"Disasters are not blessings in disguise. They are usually painful and frightening. Can we, however, find morals, lessons, and even slivers of silver linings? Of course. Do we have the capacity to survive and thrive? Yes. Do we have the capacity to grow and know when to take control, and when control is beyond us? Absolutely. Because we have the capacity to help ourselves and each other to StressRelief!"

—*Georgia Witkin, Ph.D.*

Other Newmarket Press books by Georgia Witkin, Ph.D.

The Female Stress Survival Guide
The Male Stress Survival Guide

StressRelief™
FOR DISASTERS GREAT AND SMALL

WHAT TO EXPECT AND WHAT TO DO
FROM DAY ONE TO YEAR ONE AND BEYOND

Georgia Witkin, Ph.D.

Newmarket Press • New York

This book is published in the United States of America.

First Edition

10 9 8 7 6 5 4 3 2 1

Library of Congress Cataloging-in-Publication Data
Witkin, Georgia.
    StressRelief for disasters great and small : what to expect and what to do
from day one to year one and beyond / Georgia Witkin.— 1st ed.
        p. cm.
    ISBN 1-55704-529-1
  1. Stress management. 2. Stress (Psychology)—Prevention. 3.
Relaxation. I. Title: Stress relief. II. Title.
    RA785 .W584 2002
    155.9'042—dc21

                                        2002003345

ISBN 1-55704-529-1

QUANTITY PURCHASES

Companies, professional groups, clubs, and other organizations may qualify
for special terms when ordering quantities of this title. For information, write
Special Sales Department, Newmarket Press, 18 East 48th Street, New York,
NY 10017; call (212) 832-3575; fax (212) 832-3629; or e-mail
mailbox@newmarketpress.com.

www.newmarketpress.com

Manufactured in the United States of America.

Contents

StressRelief

Introduction

On the morning of September 11, 2001, I was driving down Fifth Avenue in New York City and thinking about the patients I was scheduled to see that day, when I realized that smoke was rising up far downtown. Stopped at a red light, I could hear pedestrians talking to each other, saying a plane had accidentally crashed into the World Trade Center.

Horrified, I wondered how this could happen, and I was praying that there were no casualties when I entered my office to hear the phone ringing. It was my daughter. She was crying, and so was her baby son in her arms. She told me she had just seen a second plane fly directly into the World Trade Center, and that television reports were calling the hits "terrorism." She was crying, she said, for the victims, for her friends and her husband's friends who worked in the buildings, for our safety, and for her son's future.

This was not my daughter's first life trauma. Her son needed lifesaving surgery when he was just five weeks old and then constant care during his successful recovery. But this was her first national disaster, and far sooner than I, she realized how much this trauma would change all our lives. "What are we going to do?" she asked me. "How do we live with this?" I was in shock, but I knew the answer. "We'll figure it out," I said. "We're built to survive."

By that evening, I was on the air for the FoxNews Channel and saying it again: "We're built for emotional survival." I am even more sure of that statement now than when I first made it. I saw over the following months that every stress response serves a function, no matter how strange it may seem at first. Shock and numbness buffer our fear and permit us to function on automatic pilot in the first hours of a trauma. Hypervigilance keeps us on alert until the danger has passed. Flashbacks remind us of dangers that may return. Day by day, week by week, and month by month, we review, rework, and recover.

Over the next four months, I interviewed survivors and families of those who did not survive. I took calls from viewers and held the hands of shell-shocked private patients. I spoke to the firefighters and police whom I taught for fourteen years at Westchester Community College in the Criminal Justice Department, and met with and surveyed more than 1,000 New York City educators. As Director of The Stress Program at Mount Sinai Medical Center in New York, I worked with those suffering from nightmares, flashbacks, social withdrawal, anxiety, and depression. As contributor to the FoxNews Channel, I covered the psychology of terrorism, survivors' guilt, children's fears, and mourners' pain, and I answered questions like: "How can we tell when the normal becomes abnormal or even worse?," "When should we worry?," and "How do we know what's coming next?" As a psychiatry professor, I taught medical students why talk is so important for healing and why it takes two years for the brain to absorb losses. As a researcher, I uncovered many myths about Post-Traumatic Stress Disorder and came to see that there is a Sequence of Recovery after a disaster, but that the sequence is *not* set in stone! But most important, as a therapist, I discovered that personal tragedies can trigger similar types of reactions as a national tragedy and are often felt even more profoundly.

Soon after the terrorist attacks of September 11, 2001, Dr. Caroll Hankin, Superintendent of Schools for Syosset, Long Island, asked me to conduct a StressRelief workshop for the 1,500 employees in her school district. As a group, they were not only in shock and grieving for the many neighbors and loved ones who were lost in the devastation, but they were trying to comfort their students and help them deal with fear, anger, and confusion. We filled two auditoriums and, after a commemorative service, a live speakerphone call to the group from Senator Hillary Clinton, and four choruses of "God Bless America," we got down to work. Many spoke, many cried, and we even found that many could still laugh. Stress myths were busted, StressRelief was explained, and Emotional CPR, as described in the chapters to come, was assigned. Together we practiced some StressRelief Prescriptions on the spot.

Then the group was asked to write down the most stressful

experience they had lived through before the terrorist attacks of September 11, 2001. Next, on a personal stress scale that runs from one (lowest stress) to ten (highest stress), they were asked to rate that experience. Finally, they were asked to rate the terrorist attacks on the same personal stress scale. You may want to try this exercise yourself before you read on.

The results were a great surprise to the researchers at The Stress Program, my producers at FoxNews Channel, Dr. Hankin, and me. Although the terrible terrorist trauma received very high stress ratings, the personal traumas and losses received even higher stress ratings! Was your result the same? Here's a summary of the findings:

The most frequently mentioned personal disaster was loss of a parent or loved one. Twenty-five percent of both men and women said this had been the most traumatic personal experience of their lives so far and gave it an average of 9.2 stress points out of a possible 10. Since stress increases as our sense of control, sense of choice, and ability to predict what's coming next decreases, this is not surprising. The death of a parent or loved one usually changes our entire world. But what about 9/11? When compared to the loss of a parent, the stress rating for the disaster that had brought us together was high—but not as high. It was 7.8 stress points.

The next personal trauma listed most frequently by both men and women was divorce. Again, it's easy to understand why divorce is so traumatic since, even when we want it, the process changes our social, financial, sexual, and emotional life. And remember, as our ability to predict what's coming next decreases, stress increases. But doesn't a national disaster like a terrorist attack that changes our sense of security and safety forever sound like a stressful event, too? Of course. But, once again, not as stressful as a personal disaster. The events of September 11 received 8 stress points, but divorce received 9.2 points.

The pattern continued. Women listed illness of a parent next, and both men and women listed illness of a child. The worrying, watching, and waiting for the recovery of loved ones received, on average, 9 stress points; the worrying, watching, and waiting for the recovery of our national security received, on average, 8 points. Some listed ending a relationship, personal illness, or raising children as their most stressful experience. In each case, the stress rating for 9/11 and its fallout fell short. Only when financial problems were compared to the terrorist attacks did the national emergency receive a higher personal stress rating.

What does this mean? Does it mean that we're overly absorbed in our personal troubles or too selfish to care about the country as a whole? No. It means that we're built to love and protect those closest to us, and that it is their loss that affects us most profoundly. It means that if we can save our children, protect our parents or partners or pets, or hold on to our friends, we feel that we can survive anything. It is our involvement in the lives of those closest to us that pulls us back into daily life after a natural disaster or national crisis and helps us seek StressRelief. It is this caring for our friends and family that gives us empathy for the losses of others and leads us to charity, patriotism, and acts of heroism.

Although this book is about disasters great and small, it's now clear that there are no small disasters if the loss is personal. But we have the capacity to find StressRelief day by day if we know the way, and this book can help—from day one of a trauma to year one and beyond.

This book is dedicated to all those who have asked me to put my discoveries, information, and advice on paper. My profits from this book will go to The Stress Program at the Mount Sinai Medical Center and other charities that offer StressRelief to victims of disasters great and small.

Chapter One

Day One

We are built for disaster. We are also built for births and deaths and work and anniversaries and holidays and relocations. We humans have lived with danger since we first walked upright and formed villages that needed protection, and we have natural inborn capacities for coping with that danger. The coping, however, comes at a high cost—worth the price if it saves our lives, but too costly to overuse or abuse. We must learn to appreciate it and preserve it. And the first step is to understand it.

THE DISASTER RESPONSE

Disasters come in many sizes. The disaster response does not. Our body reacts to a tire blowing out in the same way it reacts to a building blowing up. The reaction is called the *fight-or-flight response*, or stress response, and it's a set of automatic biobehavioral changes that prepare us for the unexpected, for the uncontrollable, and the unwelcome—great or small. Here's how it works...

When a disaster hits, the brain goes on alert, and the right hemisphere starts producing quick, nonverbal reactions to the emergency. The very logical and verbal left hemisphere will deal with the meaning of the disaster later. For now, the goal is to fight or escape—the goal is survival. Our senses become more acute, and information related to our personal survival is quickly processed by the brain. Next, distress messages travel from the nervous system command center, the brain, to the body via three pathways:

1. Messages travel from the brain to the interior of the adrenal gland, which releases adrenaline into the bloodstream as a general stimulant. The result: instant readiness for fight or flight.

2. Messages travel from the brain to the autonomic nervous system, raising blood pressure, heart rate, and blood sugar levels and releasing reserves of red blood cells needed for carrying oxygen to muscles—again, preparing us for fight or flight.

3. Messages travel from the brain through motor nerves to arm, leg, and other skeletal muscles, tensing them and preparing them to carry out fight or flight—even if neither is a real possibility.

Numb and Dumb

In fact, during a disaster, the brain and body are so busy with the emergency preparations for fight or flight that there is little perception of pain or fright. Instead of responding to physical injuries with the heightened sensitivity you might expect in high-alert mode, we are more likely to be numb. A terrified victim clamped between a lion's jaws may actually feel very little because the brain has neutralized the pain message to increase the chances of clear thinking.

As for our emotions, the interplay of our nervous and endocrine systems during a disaster also leads to a counterintuitive result. People very often find that though they think they would scream during a crisis, cry out if they saw a car coming at them, or weep uncontrollably on a hijacked plane, they do not. We become dumb, which in this case means speechless. Far from stupid, this kind of dumbness is a brilliant survival reaction. Perhaps you have heard stories of the uncanny silence in the World Trade Center stairwells as the workers filed out—one of the most orderly evacuations of all time. The same survival instinct that causes the body to go on alert also subdues the emotions . . . because how can we rescue ourselves if we are weeping? How can we hear life-saving information if we are filling the air with our own noise?

If tears do flow, they are tears of fear that come from wide-open eyes as we continue to watch and listen for vital survival clues and cues around us. This laser-like attention to information that can help us is probably a descendant of an ancient instinct to be silent, an almost universal reaction that initially helped lost children be quiet so they would not attract wild animals. And it is part of the same instinct that leads us to freeze when we see danger coming, so the danger will not see us. We may not have fangs, wings, claws, odor sacs like skunks, or an ink supply like squid to help us survive, but we do have brains that make us the most adaptable species on earth.

HIGHLY SUGGESTIBLE

As much as we may be independent thinkers in our daily lives, in an emergency we have a natural tendency to follow a leader. The leader may be someone we see as an expert—someone familiar with the situation, someone who has information about an escape route, someone who has a better view of the situation than we do, or simply the person taking charge. Of course, this can lead to hysteria if those with the loudest voices are panicked or not qualified to lead, or if we think that only a few can escape.

But, more often, this suggestibility saves lives and creates heroes. In fact, it's our follow-the-leader tendency that usually accounts for the breathtaking way in which people in an emergency will band together, help each other, and become part of a working team instead of a stampede. It also explains why people who find themselves on the sidewalk in front of a burning building often cannot tell a reporter how they got there. Remember, survival hormones quickly shut down the talkative left hemisphere of the brain, which specializes in language and logic, and increase awareness in the right hemisphere, the nonverbal side. It is only later, out of danger and at leisure, that the left hemisphere analyzes the meaning of the events of recent hours, whether it is the loss of a loved one or the loss of a way of life, and gives them words.

THE PHYSICAL FORECAST FOR DAY ONE

It may take seconds, a few minutes, or several hours, but shock follows a disaster—and the shockwaves are physical, intellectual, and emotional. Let's start with their effect on your body. You've been geared up for fight or flight all day and probably did neither: no fight, no flight. If so, the adrenaline has been pouring out with nowhere to take you and all nonemergency body systems are on standby. You're likely to have a queasy stomach since digesting a grilled cheese sandwich is not a priority right now. You're likely to have a headache since your blood pressure is up in order to increase the circulation of nutrients to the muscles and oxygen to the brain. You're likely to feel dizzy or spacey or short of breath since you are probably panting without realizing it. And your chest may feel tight from working your diaphragm muscles so hard.

THE PSYCHOLOGICAL OUTLOOK FOR DAY ONE

Although seconds after a disaster hits all our reactions become heightened, in the hours after a tragedy or disaster, an emotional numbness (very much like the physical numbness we feel at the time of injury) sets in. Instead of suffering the excruciating emotional pain we might expect, we often go numb instead and feel very little. This is an innate survival mechanism. So don't feel alarmed or guilty if you're not grieving or crying, even after a great loss. Your emotions are getting a short-term rest before the long run.

THE MYTH OF THE NEAT STAGES

Now for a vital warning: if your phases and stages do not coincide precisely with those just described here or those to come, this is no cause for alarm either. In the course of counseling disaster survivors, my colleagues and I have made a surprising discovery:

- Though there may be a blueprint for post-disaster reactions, they are not carved in stone or invariable. We all move at different rates during recovery and can experience more than one symptom, even experience more than one stage, at the same time, particularly if we are in recovery from one disaster when another hits.
- What we bring to the disaster—a cool head, resilience,

vulnerability, an intact support system, experience, special-
ized knowledge, training—makes some degree of difference. A history of being overwhelmed by disaster when you
were a child, for example, may mean you still use those
childlike coping tools that worked for you back then. Or a
current health problem or death in the family may mean
your response to a disaster great or small is particularly
exaggerated.

How you enter a disaster then will influence the symptoms
you take out of it. So watch yourself with interest and make
course corrections along the way, particularly if you seem to be
stuck in a reaction and heading in the direction of trouble at work
or at home. Every symptom described so far is meant to serve a
survival function in a specific situation, but in excess or over too
long a time they can cause destructive wear and tear on you and
on those around you. Minimizing and repairing the effects of
wear and tear are the aims of the StressRelief Prescriptions.

SEEING IS BELIEVING

For the last several decades, many of us have wondered if over-
exposure to violence in the media has desensitized us and made
us less compassionate toward disaster victims and more accept-
ing of devastation and violence as a way of life. Recent terrorist
attacks and disasters have shown us that it has not! In fact,
researchers at Stanford University find that viewing a real disas-

ter on television or hearing radio bulletins as it happens live can be as alarming as being there and can trigger many of the same reactions. Even watching a videotape replay of a real disaster, like the terrorists' attacks on the World Trade Center and the Pentagon, can arouse our fight-or-flight response and plunge us into shock.

Furthermore, watching a disaster unfold from a distance may have a serious recovery disadvantage: the fight-or-flight response means we are ready to battle bad guys or flee the scene, but we have nowhere to go and no one to fight. We stay glued to the television set, and as we sit still on our couch, watching and listening, it seems as though the disaster is reoccurring every time it is replayed and the adrenaline affects us for hours, weeks, months, and perhaps even years.

EMOTIONAL CPR FOR DAY ONE

There is a widely held myth that our thoughts and behaviors are always the result of our feelings and this is a one-way process. First, we feel frightened, the myth goes, and then we think and act frightened. Fortunately, the truth is that this process can work in reverse as well, and our feelings can be the *result* of our thoughts and behaviors, not only the cause. That means we can choose our thoughts and behaviors, and therefore create the feelings of our choice. This means although a disaster may unfold in a way that leaves us feeling like a helpless victim, that feeling does not have to last long. We can change that feeling by changing our thoughts and behaviors. I call this Emotional CPR (Cognitive/ Psychological Resuscitation).

Begin this way: from minute one of Day One, select your thoughts wisely. Affirm your ability to think through problems and assure yourself that you can deal with disaster. Although those around you may try to reassure you, studies tell us that the voice we listen to most attentively is our own voice. So give yourself encouraging words and create the thoughts from which you want your feelings to flow.

StressRelief Prescriptions for Day One

Rx: Practice StressRelief Breathing. If your thinking is unclear, if shock is interfering with your ability to decide what to do next, or if you feel dizziness or other mild physical discomforts, force yourself to breathe slowly, gently, and in rhythm from the belly (not the chest), pausing after each breath. This is the way babies breathe when they are sleeping.

The reason we need lessons in this diaphragmatic breathing now is that under disaster circumstances we automatically breathe rapidly, which pushes carbon dioxide (CO_2) out of our lungs more quickly than normal. This hyperventilation may seem useful at first, since CO_2 is the waste product of respiration, but this molecule does double duty. It is the collection of carbon dioxide in the bloodstream that is the signal to the brain that it's time to take the next breath. Not enough CO_2 because you've expelled so much? No need to take a breath, responds the brain. Soon you may feel shortness of breath, dizziness, weakness, tingling fingertips and lips, and sweating. For some people, these symptoms are so uncomfortable that they create panic, and that in turn makes the symptoms worse.

You can usually stop the "panic attack" within twenty seconds to a minute by breathing slowly and pausing after every breath until the CO_2 builds up again and clear thinking returns. If you know you tend to pant or hyperventilate under stress, or if you do not know you tend to do it but experience the symptoms often, try this quick fix: Keep a small plastic bag with you and breathe into and out of it when you feel short of breath. This will quickly increase your CO_2 level.

Then you can begin the StressRelief Breathing to clear your head. Practice now—in line at the market, in the doctor's waiting room, or during a long elevator ride.

- Count back from ten to one, and take a gentle breath on each count. Let the air fill your belly, not your chest, when you breathe in. Then gently exhale, relax, and pause a beat. Try to relax more and more on each count. This is how babies breathe when they are sleeping, and it signals the brain to lower its emergency-readiness level.
- When you've become practiced, do a second set with your eyes closed, if possible. Or pretend that every time you

16

exhale your breath is a mist of your favorite color so that you create more and more of a mist of this color. The imagery will involve your right hemisphere and give you some relief from worrying, which is centered in your left hemisphere.

Rx: Try Progressive Muscle Relaxation. You can use the suggestibility, which is heightened during stressful times, to your advantage to create what Dr. Herbert Benson of Harvard University called the "Relaxation Response" with this Progressive Muscle Relaxation prescription. Some of my patients make a tape of their own voices giving the following Progressive Muscle Relaxation instructions:

1. Starting with the toes, relax them.
2. Then the feet and ankles: relax.
3. Then the calves: relax.
4. The knees: relax.
5. The thighs: relax.
6. The buttocks: relax.
7. The abdomen and stomach: relax.
8. The back and shoulders: relax.
9. The hands: relax.
10. The forearms: relax.
11. The upper arms: relax.

12. The neck: relax.
13. The face: relax.
14. Now, drift off.

You can also begin to counteract tension with the following technique: First slowly contract and relax each part of your body for ten seconds each. Then contract, then relax each part of your body more quickly to become aware of the tension/relaxation contrast.

Rx: Accept your emotions. Whatever your emotions are in the first hours after a disaster, accept them. You have enough to worry about without having to worry that your reactions are a problem! According to many researchers, 90 percent of us will begin to feel stressed or shocked by the end of Day One. Ninety percent is most but not all of us. Some may bypass shock altogether (often those trained for emergencies), while others will feel stress long before the end of Day One. All are normal reactions to an abnormal situation. Whatever your first reaction, observe it with interest and try to figure out how it may be protecting you from thoughts and feelings you cannot absorb just yet.

Rx: Know that StressRelief takes time. Soon after the first shockwave of the disaster response has crested and passed, there may be smaller second and third waves—or more disasters that start up our reactions all over again. Remember that our brain can only process new information so fast, and each of us will work through our thoughts and emotions at our own personal pace. Let the StressRelief start today... and tomorrow you will add to that foundation of feeling and healing.

Chapter Two

The First Night

As Day One becomes The First Night, we gradually lose the light, an important cue for our emotional and cognitive clocks, as well as our biological one. We shouldn't be surprised if we become disoriented, have trouble sensing the time passing, or feel more isolated. The withdrawal that felt like a choice by day seems more like a sentence by night, especially if we've lost somebody we loved.

And the fight-or-flight hormone, adrenaline, is still with us. Not only is our evening ritual disrupted or destroyed, but every effort we make to sleep or eat normally is disrupted by the influence of that adrenaline, which was present in such quantities earlier in the day that we're still feeling its stimulating effect. We are hypervigilant, hyperventilating, and hyperactive. We jump at every loud or unexpected sound, breathe rapidly until our mouths dry and our fingers tingle, and jiggle our legs and drum our fingers—even if we are immobilized on the couch. These ancient stress responses actually helped our ancestors stay ready for fight or flight through the long, dark night, but now we need sleep. We may not be able to think down our adrenaline levels yet, but we can become more comfortable with our responses as the evening comes. Rather than let these responses overwhelm us, we can observe them, understand them, and use them to reassure ourselves that we are programmed for survival.

THE PHYSICAL FORECAST FOR THE FIRST NIGHT

Hyperventilation and hyperactivity are two of a trio of disaster responses that make us feel uncomfortably nervous and wary on The First Night after a disaster, but actually they are all inborn survival capacities.

HYPERVENTILATION

During the night after the day of a disaster, the respiratory system is on alert, a condition we called hyperventilation in Chapter One. We may not be able to control the high adrenaline level that causes hypervigilance, but we can control the less-than-optimal breathing patterns that lead to hyperventilation with the StressRelief Breathing also described in Chapter One.

Remember, when we are under stress, we begin to breathe rapidly to prime ourselves for running or fighting. Soon we can get a plunge in our blood levels of carbon dioxide, the byproduct of respiration that also signals us to take the next breath. When we don't take that breath, we may begin to feel our breathing rhythm disrupted, our lips go numb, our fingertips tingle, and we become lightheaded or dizzy. This can lead to a panic attack that magnifies all of the symptoms above! Chest pains and shortness of breath may convince us we're having a heart attack—though it's more likely to be a panic attack from your hyperventilation.

Fortunately, we can bring our respiration rate back to normal with StressRelief Breathing (see Chapter One), or by breathing into and out of a small paper or plastic bag held tightly around our nose and mouth to capture the carbon dioxide we exhale and reintroduce it into the bloodstream. If we don't slow the hyperventilation ourselves, our body takes care of the problem: We get so dizzy we have to sit down and start breathing more slowly or, ultimately, we pass out—which will restore regular breathing immediately! So, take control and try StressRelief Breathing instead.

HYPERACTIVITY

Hyperactivity is the second psychophysiological state that usually makes The First Night difficult. Just as hyperventilation means the respiratory system is in overdrive, hyperactivity means the muscles are in overdrive. Fueled by adrenaline and ready for fight or flight, they're powered up and prepared to propel us out of harm's way . . . except that the disaster is often over. If we use that adrenaline after the disaster to clean up debris, board up windows, help the injured, or load the car for a trip, the hyperactivity comes in handy. But suppose we've been sitting at the kitchen table all day mourning the pet that the police took away this morning after it was hit by a car, or we haven't left the couch from the time we first saw the hurricane or crash or terrorist attack on TV. We still have adrenaline surging through our systems. This is why our legs are nervously bouncing up and down, our toes are wiggling, and our fingers are drumming. We may even shiver or shake.

As much as the voluntary muscles we use for fight or flight may be in overdrive and twitching, our smooth, involuntary muscles which control functions that are not fight-or-flight priorities are also affected. Digestion is a prime example. Since digesting a grilled cheese sandwich is not of primary importance during fight or flight, the contractions of the muscles of the intestine are also not a priority during times of high stress. The intestines, therefore, may lose their rhythm or even come to a grinding halt. The food we force ourselves to eat or eat compulsively during Day One may feel like a lump in our stomach during The First Night. Or the contractions may speed up to achieve evacuation, causing diarrhea. As the cranial vagus nerves, which run from the head to the chest and abdomen, signal the stomach to produce more acid, "butterflies" may fill our stomach, we may feel a "sinking" feeling, or have Day One of acid reflux. For all forms of hyperactivity on The First Night, use StressRelief Breathing as a slow-down signal for your body, and follow up with the Emotional CPR and StressRelief Prescriptions at the end of this chapter.

THE PSYCHOLOGICAL OUTLOOK FOR THE FIRST NIGHT

Most of us will spend this first night not only hyperventilating and hyperactive, but also reliving the dreadful events of the day. It's almost inevitable. It's the third of the trio of The First Night disaster responses. It's called hypervigilance. If the danger hasn't passed as the sun sets, hypervigilance is meant to help us stand guard through the night. Even if the immediate danger has passed, hypervigilance is meant to heighten our awareness of the possible medical or emotional needs of those around us. Bottom line: Hypervigilance will make falling alseep, and staying asleep, very difficult.

HYPERVIGILANCE

Stress puts our brains on alert. Extreme stress, like a personal betrayal, unexpected illness, or the terrorist attacks of September 11, puts our brain on highest alert. This state of stress-readiness is called hypervigilance. It is a psychophysiological term that means we are not only ready for any emergency, but we are *expecting* another emergency. Because the adrenaline from hours earlier is still circulating in our systems, our startle response is exaggerated—we jump every time the phone rings and turn our head sharply toward any movement we see out of the corner of our eye. This produces more adrenaline in a cycle that will take hours—even days—to run its course.

Hypervigilance, then, is why we won't fall asleep the minute our head hits the pillow and instead may lie awake staring at the ceiling . . . or we may go to sleep now but wake in the middle of the night at the slightest sound of traffic or a bedmate's tossing and turning. These awakenings are especially likely every hour and a half, when our sleep cycle brings us just below conscious awareness. If we don't awaken at this point from stimuli in our nighttime environment, we may wake from nightmares as we try to digest what happened on Day One. Adrenaline surges may awaken us again early in the morning—perhaps very early, before dawn—and there we are, unable to get back to sleep.

A handful of us, however, will have the opposite response, which is why I say that "neat stages" are a myth! Some, especially those who had to deal with traumas when they were very young, may find they are more likely to fall heavily asleep when they're traumatized—a condition called "somnambulistic withdrawal." When they were children, sleep may have been their only escape from stress; it worked then and is automatic now. But don't confuse somnambulistic withdrawal with relaxation, callousness, or effective StressRelief. It's a short-term emergency reaction like shock or denial, and digesting the disaster still waits in the near future.

Remember, hypervigilance may make us feel uncomfortably nervous and wary, but it's a basic survival response to disaster.

STUCK IN THE MODE

Hypervigilance, hyperventilation, and hyperactivity are all normal for The First Night, and though they may make us uncomfortable, we can reassure ourselves that they are temporary—because the brain and body simply can't stay in high gear indefinitely. For now, use the StressRelief Prescriptions below to make The First Night more bearable, more restful, and to start building a StressRelief regimen for the days to come.

EMOTIONAL CPR FOR THE FIRST NIGHT

Remind yourself that although your emotions can influence your thoughts and behaviors, the reverse is also true and you can use this information to your advantage. You can choose your thoughts and behaviors and influence your emotions. This is what I'm calling Emotional CPR, and here's the amazing part. If others tell us that things could be worse and that we are strong, it's generally ineffective as a stress-reliever. But if we say the very same things to ourselves, it is generally dramatically effective and our mood and behavior changes for the better.

For example, use the aftermath of the attacks of September 11, 2001, as a lesson in kindness, generosity, and forward motion. Few disasters, great or small, are without such lessons. Make your own list, or review mine, to help you restore some balance to your view of the world. Remember, what we choose to think about can significantly increase or decrease our stress level! Here's what I choose to think about:

- Rescue workers traveled thousands of miles to volunteer their help free of charge. They then willingly stood in line for hours waiting for their assignments.
- So much donated food and clothing poured into New York that rescue workers couldn't use it all, and some of it had to be warehoused.
- Millions of Americans donated so much blood that the Red Cross had to throw away one pint out of every five.
- Americans gave $1.2 billion to charities formed to help disaster victims and their families.
- Strangers held hands and sang together at candlelight vigils across the country.
- Relationships were rekindled as we looked up old friends to ask if they were okay.
- And business at one New York area dating service doubled as singles began to realize how much can happen in a day.

STRESSRELIEF PRESCRIPTIONS FOR THE FIRST NIGHT

For The First Night, you can reuse all of the StressRelief Prescriptions from Day One and add the following:

Rx: Make a List.
1. Pull out a pencil and make list of what has to be done in the morning to deal with the disaster.
2. Add everything that didn't get done today because of the disaster.
3. Add items for the following day and for the first week.

This simple list will help you focus on the near future, ground yourself with a plan, replace the sense of uselessness with a sense of purpose, and remind yourself that you have a "village brain"— that you are a needed member of a family and larger community. After all, one reason you are suffering now is that you care for others. They care for you, too!

Rx: Do something physical.
If you are hyperactive and overenergized, you'll need to get rid of some of that adrenaline before you can truly rest. Run around the house or block until you have used up some of the adrenaline and feel your energy level come down or until you have to stop! Or put on music with a beat faster than your heartbeat, about seventy-two beats per minute, and run in place. Or really dance to the music or jump rope or march or even paint a wall—as long as the movement is rhythmic and rigorous, you'll be able to relax once the adrenaline has burned off.

Rx: Take one task at a time.
Your concentration probably isn't very good right now, and trying to do more than one task at a time

may mean you start everything and finish nothing. This will only increase your sense of frustration and increase your stress levels. Choosing one job and making a little progress, on the other hand, will help to restore your sense of control.

Rx: Bore yourself to sleep. If you can't sleep because your brain is on alert, one way to find StressRelief from hypervigilance is to flood your brain with the predictable. Follow your regular bed-time routine so you know exactly what's coming next. Turn on your favorite music so you know every note that's coming. Rock yourself like a baby so your body can predict every motion. And then lull your brain to sleep with easy, repetitive prayers, poems, nursery rhymes, or even by counting sheep. The familiar words and repeated rhythms help to quiet the stress response. If you awaken during the night, try once again reciting a prayer, poem, or comforting phrase or mantra. Soothing thoughts do soothe the emotions.

Rx: Reach out. Our sense of isolation increases with the darkness, so don't wait too long to call a friend, relative, or counselor. Though the television seems like a friendly presence, its images have the power to cause pain, and it will never respond to you. However, real people—face to face—will. They will help you feel more connected, listen to your thoughts and fears, and share your concerns.

Chapter Three

The Day After

The world we live in is full of disasters large and small—from floods to failed tests, from major military wars to petty wars of words, and from losses in the stock market to the loss of a favorite doll. Fortunately, we have many capacities to help us deal with them all, and most of the time it's with a flexibility and resourcefulness that can surprise even ourselves. Our resourcefulness and flexibility may temporarily fail us, however, during the moments after we awake on The Day After a disaster. In those moments, we are newly accosted by our sudden memory of what happened just yesterday. On this first morning, for a few moments, we are likely to hope and pray that the disaster was just a nightmare. But soon we are reminded of the reality that we'll be living with from this day on.

A DAY OF CONFLICTS

Of all the days in a disaster aftermath, The Day After is also the most confusing. No matter what kind of disaster it was, our research shows that about 90 percent of us continue to feel stressed on the second day. That stress takes many forms. To the mix of numbness, dumbness, hypervigilance, hyperactivity, hyperventilation, and disorientation of the last twenty-four hours we may add waves of emotional pain, distrust, irritability, fear, or fatigue. We may feel lucky to be alive but at the same time guilty to be alive; activated by the adrenaline rush but at the same time helpless and mentally exhausted; angry but at the same time numb and immobilized; and, therefore, very confused.

As if this weren't enough to deal with, we start seeing instant replays of the disaster on television, if the disaster was national—or in our mind's eye, if it was personal. Either way, sights, sounds, and emotions will intrude at unexpected times all day as our brain tries again and again to digest the shocking news. We'll go over it and over it as we try to desensitize ourselves, process the information, and prepare for what comes next.

VIEWERS' STRESS

Are you wondering why television viewers are so affected by disasters like the Oklahoma City bombing, the Columbine shootings, and of course, the Pentagon and the World Trade Center attacks, even though they witnessed the disaster from miles away, safe in their living rooms? Remember that Stanford University researchers found seeing a real-life disaster on television can have as powerful an effect on us as seeing the actual disaster.

31

After we realize that the disaster was not just Hollywood special effects, the reality of the event begins to penetrate our consciousness, and we lock into an epic struggle to understand the meaning of the event: how it affects us and our fellow human beings, how it changes us, and how it could have happened at all. If it isn't already a personal disaster, The Day After is usually the day when the body count will shift from being a number ("Scores Killed in Bomb Blast") to a collection of heartbreaking individual stories: the teen who clung to a tree for hours while flood waters raged around him, the young mother shot during a riot while nursing her baby on a stoop a block away, or the child whose father didn't come home. Because we have a "village brain" that can't really grasp huge tolls of loss but easily empathizes with individuals, their tragedy will become our tragedy.

Today we'll think about it, talk about it, and endure the terrible replays. Tonight we may have nightmares about it or lie half awake as unedited images play across our minds. Through this painful process, our brains are beginning to integrate the experience of Day One as a piece of permanent information.

THE PHYSICAL FORECAST FOR THE DAY AFTER

The Day After is not too early to begin "taking care" of yourself. Researchers find that people who suffer major disasters are more likely to experience certain health problems later on than people who did not. A Florida study, for example, finds that chronic fatigue patients who were personally affected by Hurricane Andrew in 1992 had more severe relapses than those not in the hurricane's path. Other studies suggest an increased risk of episodes of allergies, rheumatoid arthritis, ulcerative colitis, irritable bowel syndrome, or high blood pressure after a very stressful event.

This is not a reason to become alarmed or throw our hands up in resignation and head for the local bar or diner. Rather, it's a warning that we are already vulnerable to health problems after a disaster, and that reaching for comfort food, alcohol, cigarettes, and other quick fixes can make matters worse and create even more stress. It's important on The Day After to eat simply and wisely, set aside time for pauses, even if you can't rest, contact loved ones for moral support, and sleep. Finally, it's important to look inside to see what remains of the hope, purpose, and self-knowledge we had before the disaster. Just knowing they're still there—and they are—can give us a reassuring glimpse of the future.

THE PSYCHOLOGICAL OUTLOOK FOR THE DAY AFTER

Adjusting to the aftermath of a disaster is slow work, with many variations on the theme. If we feel exhausted and dull while everyone around us seems to be going about their business, we may worry that we're abnormal. We are not. If, on the other hand, we're among the lucky ones who wake up on The Day After feeling relatively whole, we also may worry that we're abnormal. We are not. But we are different. Those trained to handle disasters, such as experienced emergency personnel, bring a feeling of control to the situation, and are likely to be resilient. People with chronic physical or mental health problems, high underlying stress levels from the loss of a job, or cash flow problems or those who have recently been evicted or served with divorce papers are less likely to bounce back quickly. The same may be true of people with major disasters like the current one in their history: the terrorist attacks in New York City and Washington, D.C., triggered relapses of Post-Traumatic Stress Disorder (PTSD) in people who had been treated successfully after Oklahoma City.

EMOTIONALLY-TOXIC SHOCK

The lesson is that each of us comes to a disaster, and reacts to a disaster, with different degrees of stress. The good news is that, according to the National Center for Post-Traumatic Stress Syndrome in White River Junction, Vermont, most of us will not suffer from debilitating stress symptoms after a disaster. The bad news, however, is that some of us will suffer from an unusually intense reaction that I call *Emotionally-Toxic Shock*. This is a disaster reaction, which interferes with our normal activities to such a degree that it requires special StressRelief. Use this checklist to score the severity of your post-disaster stress reaction. Give yourself one point if the following is *sometimes* true for you, and two points if it's *usually* true for you:

EMOTIONALLY-TOXIC SHOCK CHECKLIST

___I am so tired that I can't get out of bed to do the simplest task.

___I am so tense that I can't complete most tasks I start.

___I am so distracted that I forget to eat.

___I am so numb that I stop communicating with most people around me, neither asking nor answering questions nor showing interest in conversation.

___I give quick nonverbal reactions, even to situations that need discussion or thought before action.

___I can't make most decisions.

___I can't express sympathy, even when I try.

If you have even one point on this checklist, you are suffering from some degree of shock and should try at least one of the prescriptions at the end of this chapter. If your score is above just three points, your reaction is severe, and you should be practicing many of the StressRelief Prescriptions and talking with supportive family and friends about your stress. Above five points, it's important that you speak to your family physician, religious counselor, or a mental health specialist, or the start of your recovery may be unnecessarily delayed due to shock. These professionals can help you begin to help yourself.

EMOTIONAL CPR FOR THE DAY AFTER

The fight-or-flight response is still likely to be running your life on The Day After, so it's important to pause at least five times during the day to catch your breath and review what you are thinking and doing. Since you can do much to change what you feel by changing what you think and what you do, choose to think calm thoughts and behave "as if" you are calm. The fight-or-flight response is, after all, a response and you can turn it down, or even off, by not triggering it with dire thoughts or frantic actions. Then remind yourself that what remains of the fight-or-flight response is a sign of stamina and the will to live, and take some of the steps listed below to revive yourself and get on with what you have to do today.

STRESSRELIEF PRESCRIPTIONS FOR THE DAY AFTER

For The Day After, eat nutritiously so you'll build strength for the coming days, return some calls to ensure that your support network will be in place, start making lists to regain some sense of control (and so your memory won't be overtaxed when you're so distracted), and review everything for which you are still thankful to regain some optimism or hope.

You can also use all of the prescriptions for Day One and The First Night. To these, we add:

Rx: Get out of the house. You may be tempted to unplug the phone, pull down the shades, and slide deep under the covers where the news can't find us, but consider this: though we can't do anything about the global political situation, the physical nature of the planet, or the aging process of human beings, we can help family and friends, and they can help us. Because we all have a "village brain," we do better when we see others face to face. Just as the youngest baby is programmed to smile at us and make us smile back—and form a bond—we're all programmed to take care of each other. If you don't know what to do to make yourself feel better, others may naturally have ideas for getting your daily life back to normal. If you're shell-shocked or having symptoms of Emotionally-Toxic Shock, people around you can pick up signs you can't pick up in yourself. Provide yourself with opportunities to behave normally, to reengage, and to increase your sense of control. Reach out to the people who are important in your life, share your experiences, and feel yourself reactivate in response to others.

Rx: Volunteer. If there's been a disaster and you're still on your feet, never in your life have you been more needed. Volunteering will prove that though you've had losses, you still have something to give; though you feel drained, you still have strength. And volunteering puts you in a position to socialize face-to-face with others, which is always good for everyone. Finally, volunteering helps your health: Allan Luks, author of *The Healing Power of Doing Good*, finds that people who volunteer weekly are ten times more likely to say they're healthy than people who volunteer only once a year. The volunteers report fewer headaches and backaches and less arthritis pain, possibly because nurturing behavior may flood us with endorphins, the body's natural painkillers. Luks calls the feeling we get from volunteering a "helper's high." If you can't volunteer in person, giving money to rescue efforts and disaster relief funds can give you a sense of purpose. (For more information on helping others, see Chapter Twelve.)

Rx: Get professional help. If you're feeling sad or shocked, alone, and unable to help yourself, this is not the time to tough it out. Reach for resources: friends, family, clergy, and professional counselors. By talking to others and by sharing and comparing your experiences and reactions, you may find that your thoughts are not too extreme to express after all if those around you are recommending professional help.

Chapter Four

The First Week

The First Week following a disaster is often a blend of the real and the surreal. We may go to work and pay the bills, but the trauma is never far from our minds. And that's not all bad. Even when we're not consciously dealing with the experience we've just been through, our mind is working to integrate it with all the other experiences of our lives and make some sense of it. The Myth of the Neat Stages remains the rule. We will share many common recovery experiences, but the sequence of these experiences is not invariable. And many will move at a common pace to recovery, but many will amble or race. Just the very process of observing our progress can help us understand our own recovery and feel more comfortable with it. Knowledge is power, and forewarned is forearmed.

24/7

On the day of a disaster, our brain sends urgent bulletins of danger to our muscles, heart, blood vessels, and digestive system. But the stress response that follows is not like a twenty-four-hour virus that's gone the next day. The fight-or-flight hormones keep circulating twenty-four hours a day, and the brain and body stay on alert all seven days that first week. And as the week after a disaster wears on, particularly if we have to continue to deal with any aftermath of the disaster, most of us will start to feel the effects of long-term activation of a stress defense system intended for short-term use. In fact, during the first week after the World Trade Center and Pentagon attacks, one poll reported that 70 percent of us felt depressed, 40 percent had difficulty concentrating, and 33 percent had insomnia.

THE PHYSICAL FORECAST FOR THE FIRST WEEK

Long-term stress can also produce a progression of physical side effects that begin during The First Week. As the body struggles to accommodate a stress response day after day, blood flow shifts to large skeletal muscles and decreases to the gastrointestinal tract and to the skin. The first signs of such shifts might be cold hands and feet, then gradually a pale or sallow complexion, and finally headaches or blood pressure problems. The endocrine glands react to prolonged stress, too. They cause the release of extra sugars for energy into the bloodstream, and extra insulin to break down these sugars for immediate use. If too much insulin is produced, blood sugar levels can become too low, a condition called hypoglycemia. We feel tired and reach for a cigarette, coffee, cola, or sweets to give us a lift. Then even more insulin production is stimulated, and a low blood-sugar cycle begins.

Wear and Tear Are Inevitable

Sometimes a week of stress aggravates a pre-existing condition or tendency. Think of this as wear and tear on the body's weak spots. The stress-aggravated problems below are all susceptible to flare-ups after a disaster—great or small.

- Allergies
- Irritable bowel syndrome
- High blood pressure
- Rheumatoid arthritis
- Ulcerative colitis
- Cardiac arrhythmia
- Peptic ulcer
- Hyperventilation
- Asthma
- Myocardial infarction (heart attack)
- Skin disorders

Many symptoms of stress are less serious than the problems above, but mimic serious diseases, and our anxiety about them adds more stress to an already stressful situation. I often hear patients in the midst of emotional traumas deciding that they have

a brain tumor, coronary disease, or cancer, based on some of the
following stress symptoms:

- Headaches
- Chest pains
- Nausea
- Dizziness
- Cold sweats
- Swallowing difficulties (esophageal spasms)
- Chronic fatigue
- Backaches
- Heartburn (hyperacidity)
- Urinary frequency
- Muscle spasms
- Memory impairment
- Stomach "knots" or "butterflies"
- Panic attacks
- Constipation
- Diarrhea
- Neck aches
- Insomnia

The good news is that most of these symptoms are not danger signs of serious diseases if they appear during the week following a disaster. The bad news is that they may eventually
become more serious problems:

- The stress messages that travel from the brain through motor nerves to arm, leg, and other skeletal muscles prepare us for emergencies short-term, but their long-term effect is to fatigue those muscles.
- Likewise, the stress messages that travel from the brain through autonomic nerves to the heart, lungs, intestines, sweat glands, blood vessels, liver, kidneys, endocrine glands, and other organs gear us up for fight or flight short-term, but their long-term effect is to exhaust these organs.
- And the stress messages that travel from the hypothalamus in the brain to the pituitary, and then to other glands that release hormones which raise energy production short-term, often create imbalances in the body's hormone-driven functions when they're sent 24/7, day after day, particularly in a woman's finely-tuned reproductive system, including the menstrual cycle.

And the physical changes are only half of the picture. Psychologically, a week of stress is likely to produce the Six D's.

THE PSYCHOLOGICAL OUTLOOK FOR THE FIRST WEEK

As the fatigue and exhaustion of stress overdrive take their toll, we begin to see six time-release psychological phenomena.

The Six D's

Distraction. Before a disaster, making soup in the kitchen while fixing a bicycle on the patio and checking on the game in the TV room was probably no problem—it's called multitasking. After a disaster, sticking with even a single task until the end is usually difficult. The reasons could be several:

- Thoughts of what we've just been through may keep intruding and interrupting our flow.
- The simple task we're trying to finish may seem suddenly irrelevant.
- Fatigue from the fitful sleep of last night is making it harder to focus.
- Adrenaline levels are so high that our body and brain are in fight-or-flight mode: listening for danger and ready to escape, which is not ideal for concentration.
- The brain is so busy digesting the trauma we've experienced that new information creates instant overload.

So, if that pen you had in your hand a moment ago seems to be gone from the face of the earth although you haven't left the room, don't assume it's a brain tumor or early dementia. Most likely it's distraction, and that's "normal" for the first week after a disaster.

Disorganization. Although you may be moving at 90 or 95 percent of your normal speed during the first week after a disaster, what's not getting done may include some very crucial items, and the missing 5 or 10 percent can snowball into time-wasters as you have to backtrack to clean up the mess. And don't be surprised if your sense of direction fails you when you come out of elevators or drive to the market; following directions may be even more difficult. Not only is your real world disorganized for now, but as a result your internal maps and charts are, too. Even your memories may be difficult to retrieve, and you may find that familiar names are on the tip of your tongue rather than readily available.

Depression. Our initial reaction to disasters great or small is first shock and confusion, then anxiety—and depression. This is generally not a clinical or severe depression, however. The deep sense of loss that can follow any disaster has usually not taken hold yet. Instead we feel shaken, stressed, and startled... and the mental and physical fatigue at the end of a week is closer to the blues or the blahs than a severe depression.

If a more severe depression develops, if feelings of hopelessness, worthlessness, and sleeplessness begin to run our lives; if we lose interest in sex, food, or other pleasures of life, or even life itself; and if all of the above are most intense in the morning; then, it's time to put this book down and get help immediately. Though we may believe that nothing or no one can help us, something or someone can. Underlying the feeling of depression is often anger or loss, which a therapist or counselor may be able to address with talk, medication, or both. Or the feeling of depression may be a symptom of a biochemical change caused by the stress of the disaster's aftermath. Again, supportive therapy and/or medication can help. It may be reassuring to know that not everyone is likely to develop a serious depression after a disaster. Risk factors generally include recent preceding traumas such as the loss of a parent or job, previous episodes of serious depression, or a family history, which may point to a genetic predisposition to depression.

Sometimes depression in The First Week has a very different face. Instead of feeling that we can't eat and can't sleep, all we may want to do is eat and sleep. We want to pull the covers over our heads and "not deal," as the kids say. This is when we're most at risk for self-medication attempts involving alcohol, cigarettes, caffeine, tranquilizers, and over-the-counter sleeping remedies. Again, supportive threrapy and/or short-term medication can make a difference. Don't be a victim of depression as well as a victim of disaster. Reach out for help.

Destabilization. Despite our numbness or depression, unexpected emotions often break through and make us feel off-balance or destabilized. We cry during commercials showing happy families reaching out and touching each other, and get choked up singing national anthems. We get irritated while waiting in lines and angry at slights. And these symptoms will get worse before they get better. We feel like we need emotional release and tend to find outlets any way we can, even if they are indirect, inappropriate, or aimed at the innocent.

Decision-making difficulties. The disaster that we were unable to control a few days ago is sending waves of uncertainty and confusion through us now, and as our ability to predict what's coming next drops, our stress increases even more. More stress means more distraction, disorganization, depression, and destabilization, and then decision-making difficulties begin to develop. In part, decisions are difficult because we can't predict how we're going to feel from minute to minute or day to day. In part, the difficulties reflect the ways in which the trauma has made our world less predictable. So it's 3 P.M. and we're starving but still haven't decided what to order for lunch. We've changed our clothes three times, and the outfit still seems vaguely wrong. We've scheduled evening plans and then changed our mind about keeping the plans. The big decisions can usually be postponed, but the small ones cannot—and will feel painfully difficult.

Dependency fantasies. In the days after an unpredictable event occurs, the most independent individual may have thoughts of being cared for. It would be so nice to retreat to a walled estate guarded by a security staff. It would be so nice to spend a week in the hospital for nothing too serious, turn off the phone, receive flowers from those who love us, have food brought regularly, watch television or movies all day, and be appreciated even more when we get home. These fantasies give us some imaginary and temporary relief from responsibility and take us to places where we feel safe, but then reality intrudes!

EMOTIONAL CPR FOR THE FIRST WEEK

Remember: what we think and what we do will help shape what we feel, and that's good news, because we have more control over our thoughts and behaviors than we realize. To feel a greater sense of control, choose thoughts and behaviors that reinforce your sense of control. This is what I mean by Emotional CPR.

This week, focus on what you're managing to get done; appreciate the effort you're making and let your progress be proof that you have started returning to normal. Notice the moments when you feel emotionally level, and let them be signs that you're still you.

Those who find themselves stuck in high gear can use their thoughts to guide them to a more comfortable operating mode. We can remind ourselves that this particular disaster is over now and not likely to strike twice.

Those who find they're not getting back to basics can use the "as if" technique. If we don't feel like tackling our long "To Do" list, we can behave "as if" we're motivated and energized and *do it anyway*! By behaving "as if," we're putting ourselves into situations that will help move us in that direction—we'll be with other people we wouldn't have been with otherwise, we'll be getting feedback we wouldn't have gotten otherwise, and we'll feel new demands on ourselves, which is not a bad thing because it can make us feel needed, vital, and alive. If we behave as if things are normalized, pretty soon they will be even more so.

StressRelief Prescriptions for The First Week

Rx: Take breaks. A total of twenty minutes of StressRelief a day is enough to decrease stress symptoms and improve mood, according to researchers like Herbert Benson, M.D., of Harvard University. That's a *total* of twenty minutes—two minutes of breathing exercises in a stuck elevator, four minutes of progressive muscle relaxation while waiting in a long line, or fifteen minutes of walking or meditation all count toward the total. The effect of these breaks is to help reduce adrenaline production . . . and prevent the insomnia, headaches, stomach upsets, and other disturbances that may linger for years unless we do something about them now. So, take a break.

In fact, according to many studies, hormones produced under stress can suppress the number of blood cells that protect us against infections and even cancers. This may help to explain why widows and widowers are at higher risk of illness for the first two months after the death of a spouse, and why stress precedes sore throats and colds far more frequently than it follows them.

Bottom line: We can't fight chronic stress and still fight illness efficiently. So if you think you can't afford to schedule downtime right now, consider this: Without twenty minutes of downtime a day by choice, you're likely to have more downtime later, without choice, because of stress symptoms. You'll find yourself lying in a darkened room with a migraine, lying awake at night with insomnia, or immobilized by stomachaches or back pains. Take breaks right now from rescue efforts, daily demands, or even mourning, and you'll increase your sense of control and decrease your recovery time.

Rx: Take physical care. Though many Americans began to throw caution to the winds and feast on cheesecake and wine after the terrorist attack, Bruce McEwen, Ph.D., of The Rockefeller University in New York, reminds us that this is dangerous under stressful conditions: Prolonged stress usually changes patterns of living, including eating more high-fat food, sleeping badly, skipping exercise, or drinking more, he says. These in turn cause changes in the stress hormones, which in turn increase our risk of heart disease, depression, and some types of cancer. The setting may have changed, but the risks have not! By neglecting or abusing ourselves now, we are setting ourselves up for more stress in the future. This is a time to take care of ourselves with as much care as always—maybe even more.

Rx: Plan for the Six D's. If decision-making is difficult, if you're so disorganized that order is elusive, or if you're so distracted that you forgot where you parked the car, take a breath, pause, and try again. Then, plan for next time. Write more notes to yourself, post them where you won't miss them, and expect less of yourself for now. And don't blame yourself for the Six D's. Putting yourself down won't get the e-mail done or help you find the car.

Rx: Get back to basics. Choose to get back to dealing with daily demands. Stock up, fix up, pick up, and repair. Filling the refrigerator, picking up children's clothes, or picking up a hammer restores our sense of control. We may not be able to solve the anthrax problem or prevent earthquakes, but we can clean a kitchen drawer and reorganize our wallet—and our brain reacts as if order has been brought to the world for the moment.

Getting back to basics also brings us into contact with others, and the interactions are usually reassuring. We get to see others going about daily tasks, gather information or sympathy or support, feel less isolated, and are reminded of the roles we fill and why we are needed. Going back to basics does not mean that we are disrespecting a parent who died or a colleague we lost. It means we are programmed to move out of suspended animation and take care of business to insure our own survival—not just physical survival but psychological survival as well.

Rx: Take part in ceremony and ritual. Holding candles and singing with others in a vigil, attending a "town meeting" where people can talk and cry together, presenting the monies collected in a huge fund-raiser to a recipient can bring us closer. These are also a great antidote to depression because they remind us that coming together in times of trauma is something we do naturally. Even mourning rituals, like funerals, remind us that coming together with others can give us needed closure and remind us that we are supported and cared for.

Rx: Talk. During the first week, as the shock begins to wear off, those of us who have had a direct loss—a parent, child, friend, or colleague—will be going through acute stress and grief. We will be hit over and over by waves of pain, and we may hear ourselves sighing. The world will seem unreal—and one of the best ways to reconnect is to talk, talk, talk. If there's no one to talk to, look for someone—ask for a counselor or go to religious services or family gatherings.

Why do experts advise talking after every crisis, national or personal? Because talking gives us:

- A sense of "doing" something
- An opportunity to "hear" ourselves
- A chance to "listen" to ourselves as others would
- An opportunity to adjust our thoughts and feelings
- A chance to better understand what we're thinking or feeling

Besides, most feelings are less ominous when they are said out loud to others in the light of day than when they are silently thought, alone, in the middle of the night.

Rx: Listen. If someone has had a direct loss, be ready to listen, listen, listen! Repeat back what they say so they know you heard every word and that none of them are too dreadful to be said out loud. It's wise to avoid clichés such as "I know how you feel . . ." unless you have had a similar loss and really do know! A simple "I'm sorry" tends to be what brings the most comfort to the most people. It's important to reassure all talkers that you'll be there long after the press has left and relief services have gone. Pay attention to children and the elderly since they tend to be lost in the shuffle. One might think that children wouldn't have a severe reaction since they seem to be less aware of the event; however, in my work for *KidStress*, I've seen that the cue for child stress is grown-up stress—from teachers and parents on down to older siblings. And the greater they think are their chances of losing us, the more frightened they will be. As for the elderly, we assume that because they have lived longer they're more philosophical, but their pain may be even greater if they lived through many disasters before . . . and have memories of those losses returning full force now.

Chapter Five

The First Month

At the beginning of The First Month, the disaster may still feel fresh and the symptoms raw—irritability, insomnia, disorientation, distractibility, nervousness, neediness, crying, and sighing. But by the end of The First Month, they are likely to be more muted and even familiar. A few days after the terrorist attacks of September 2001, for example, about 70 percent of respondents in one poll reported they were depressed, 40 percent had difficulty concentrating, and 33 percent had insomnia. At three weeks, however, depression was down to 42 percent, difficulty concentrating affected just 21 percent, and insomnia was a problem for only 18 percent. But progress toward StressRelief is anything but direct because the Six D's are often replaced by the Three G's—grief, guilt, and grim predictions—and they undermine our progress. Knowing what's coming can help.

GRIEF

Although there are enormous individual differences in recovery from disasters, grief reactions often share some similar elements.

Being aware of our own bereavement process will not change our mourning, but it can reassure us that our feelings are normal and will gradually evolve into reengagement with the life around us.

Grief Element 1: Escape. If grief feels overwhelmingly painful, attempts to escape are natural. The simplest maneuver is to try to avoid any thought or mention of the loss. For a while, some will go on "automatic pilot"—act as if nothing has happened, and attend to business and continue work. Some may withdraw from friends, family, and work to avoid mention of or association with memories. And some may become temporarily numb and unfeeling.

Grief Element 2: Magical thinking. Attempts to keep loved ones we lost alive by "seeing" and "hearing" them is not uncommon, nor are beliefs that they are still right here on earth in spirit. Or we may try to substitute someone to take the role of the deceased. These beliefs and behaviors themselves are not a problem and may even be part of a long-held faith. They only become a problem if our initial loss isn't confronted. Then mourning will continue and often interfere with new relationships.

Grief Element 3: Sadness and despair. The "work" of grief is to eventually deal with the reality of a loss or losses, and when the reality begins to settle in, despair may become an element of grief. The turning point will be a change of focus—from helplessness with regard to the disaster to power and control with regard to our own lives. The choices and changes we begin to make, or are forced to make as time goes by, will begin re-engagement.

Grief Element 4: Recovery and relief. Although there are many recovery patterns, in my clinical experience, I've noticed one common characteristic: the survivor's healthy sense of surprise that he or she has been able to begin to manage loss and grief at some point, and perhaps even forget the disaster for moments at a time. Often that point comes during The First Month, as friends and family usually rally and talk, vent, and comfort each other. In fact, by the end of The First Month, the world expects survivors to get on with it—and makes demands. The expectations may be premature and naïve, but the effect is to move recovery along. At the end of four weeks, the brain is getting used to the idea that there has been a disaster and the body is getting tired of being on alert morning, noon, and night. But the beginning of recovery and StressRelief may also mean some guilt.

GUILT

When StressRelief and recovery finally begin, very often, so does guilt: "How quickly I forget!" or "How could I have enjoyed that movie after such a disaster?" or "I thought I'd never get over the loss…" Even though in our instant-gratification culture we want everything within seconds, including our own recovery, and even though others may expect us to recover far too quickly, we still tend to feel startled when we actually do begin to recover. And if lives were lost, the astonishment often becomes what's called *survivor guilt.* As the days go by and we astonish ourselves by taking care of business and those who need us, we tell ourselves we're doing very well. Others pat us on the back and say the same. But then there's the guilt, especially in the morning: "If I'm doing so well, then why is the dawn so gray?"

Here's why the dawn is gray: Although about 90 percent of Americans find themselves back in the swing of their daily routine in the first month, it's likely to be two full years before we automatically remember the disaster first thing in the morning; until then, we must go through the painful process of waking up and having the memory intrude later. If we grew up with Mom always being there, if we went to the same office every weekday for twenty years, or if we always saw the World Trade Center out the window, that's part of our brain's expectation. We will be startled by any change—sometimes forever. This is why we're surprised to see clear skin in the mirror even though it has been ten years since our acne went away and why people who lived through the Depression still fear being poor. When there's a national or personal loss, the brain will have to remind itself many times of the new information before it's reconfigured to reflect our new situation.

GRIM PREDICTIONS

It takes emotional strength to be optimistic about the future in hard times—and it takes a kind of physical recuperation, too. Though negativity and hopelessness about the future may seem to be psychological problems, their origin is partly biochemical too. Not only does our adrenaline level naturally drop in the first weeks after a disaster, so does our serotonin level, a brain chemical that helps us stay calm and ward off depression, tension, anger, confusion, sadness, and fatigue. The more extended the stress, the more our serotonin is used up and the more depressed we're likely to become. Reasoning with ourselves and talking with friends, family, or a therapist can actually influence our brain biochemistry. (See Emotional CPR below.) A number of different prescription antidepressants can do the same, especially the newer class of *selective serotonin reuptake inhibitors* (SSRIs). Consult your physician for more information.

THE PHYSICAL FORECAST FOR THE FIRST MONTH

By now, anyone who watches television news or reads newspapers is familiar with the term Post-Traumatic Stress Disorder (PTSD) described by the National Institute of Mental Health as a debilitating condition that follows a terrifying event. We associate the terms with frightening psychological symptoms like emotional numbness, sleep problems, depression, or being easily startled. We do not, in general, associate the condition with physical symptoms, but there are physical symptoms that often follow a terrifying event and they can begin to emerge between one and three months after the disaster. Be suspicious of any increase in the frequency of the following:

- Hand tremors, lip quivers, eyelid twitches
- Vague queasiness, gas pains, or diarrhea
- Rapid heartbeats, skipped heartbeats, slow heartbeats
- Heat waves, cold chills, or shivering
- Backaches, leg muscle cramps, neck spasms
- Acne, increased blotchiness, allergic reactions
- Bloating, swelling of legs, breast engorgement

For some, these symptoms will pass in three to six months, but others will have symptoms that last much longer and become chronic. Simple StressRelief Breathing can help since the slow, deep breaths counteract the rapid heartbeats, lightheadedness, and other symptoms of hyperventilation. And there's more help in the StressRelief Prescriptions at the end of the chapter.

THE PSYCHOLOGICAL OUTLOOK FOR THE FIRST MONTH

For some of us, the pain of the first month is so great that we look for something, *anything,* to take it away. We look for escape . . . and we may find it in several ways, which may make long-term StressRelief even more difficult:

"Undoing" fantasies. To escape from grief and other types of pain as well, some of us go back in our minds to the moments before the disaster and dwell on what could have or should have been, including what *we* could have or should have done. In our minds we prevent the disaster, save lives, or emerge unscathed as a hero. For the moment, we escape from the pain of recalling the real disaster! It works so well and is so rewarding to us that we tend to spend more and more time in fantasyland and less and less time in the real world. When our minds are busy imagining what could have been, we're avoiding scenes of what really was and exposure to the pain that will eventually help to desensitize us.

Escape eating. Once our appetite returns, we may find that we make up for lost food and rebound into eating as if there were no tomorrow! That may actually be what we believe if we're a little depressed, and if there's no tomorrow, why not eat whatever we feel like eating today? I call it "what-the-heck" eating. And then there's the special class of foods that remind us of Grandma's kitchen or our favorite small diner and lead us into "down-home eating": mashed potatoes, gravy, biscuits, cookies . . . and at least two helpings, of course. Finally, there's just plain anxiety eating: Favorite foods include cake, candy, cookies, bread, and pasta, which all, maybe not coincidentally, contain carbohydrates. Carbs are known to help increase brain serotonin, which in turn may take the edge off our depression, tension, anger, confusion, sadness, and fatigue, and give us a nice post-meal calmness. Short-term it is a small comfort; long-term it is a big mistake—physically and psychologically.

Drinking and recreational drugs. After the World Trade Center and Pentagon attacks of September 11, 2001, counseling centers reported a significant increase in the number of people needing alcohol and drug counseling. The signs of this pursuit of oblivion were at first not visible in the bars and night spots, which went empty—because people may have been doing more solo drinking and drugging at home. This is never a good pattern to establish, since at home it's easy to overdo when no one is watching. Though alcohol may help us fall asleep, it interferes with our ability to stay asleep. And perhaps more important, though drinking and drugs may dull the memory of a disaster and our anxiety, when we sober up, we've made less progress in processing information than those who did not use "anesthesia."

Tranquilizers. Three weeks after the September 2001 attacks, tranquilizer prescriptions were reported to be up 15 to 20 percent, and sleeping pill prescriptions up 20 percent. It's important to remember that when tranquilizers or sleeping pills are prescribed for disaster stress, they are literally, as well as figuratively, just a quick fix—they are safe to use for no more than two weeks. After that, it's time to re-evaluate with a physician.

DANGER SIGNS

Four weeks after the terrorists' attacks, crisis centers reported an average of thirty calls or more a day, at least half for severe anxiety. And they were glad to get those calls, because it showed people were taking action to overcome their stress reactions. How do you know whether intervention is needed? See whether the reaction is interfering with daily life. Ask yourself if your stress has led to:

- Threatened or destroyed relationships
- Neglected daily tasks and work duties
- Meaningless and directionless activities
- Overwhelming fears
- Insurmountable phobias

These are all signs that outside help is in order. If you or someone close to you has checked even one box, reach out for a crisis counselor or ask your family physician for a referral.

EMOTIONAL CPR FOR THE FIRST MONTH

As I've said in previous chapters, many of us already know that emotion can color our thinking and behavior, but thinking and behavior can also direct our emotions, and when it does, I call this process Emotional CPR, for Cognitive/Psychological Resuscitation. If in this first month your emotions seem out of control, let your brain and behavior, which you can control, lead the way.

If you're overwhelmed by phobias and irrational fears, talk to yourself using the words you imagine a logical, levelheaded friend would use: "You know it's extremely unlikely that another hurricane this destructive will come during your lifetime" and "You know it's extremely unlikely that you'll be mugged again." If a gray sky or dark street give you a sense of foreboding, observe that most of the time, gentle showers come from gray skies, and people are probably sleeping peacefully inside the homes lining dark streets. If the sound of an airplane makes you hunch your shoulders defensively, observe that the vast majority of the time, airplanes are carrying not terrorists but vacationers and business people to their destinations. This kind of talk therapy can actually begin to reverse the biochemical processes that cause fears and phobias. And remember, although these reassurances are usually not effective when we read them or hear them from others, they are breathtakingly effective when we say them to ourselves.

All of the StressRelief Prescriptions from the previous chapters of this book still work in The First Month. Now add the following:

StressRelief Prescriptions for The First Month

Rx: Get help with substance problems. When drinking, drugs, and eating become out of control—you can use their effect on your daily life as a gauge—stop them before they do more damage and cause more stress. One way is to crowd them out using other ways to feel better, such as these prescriptions.

Rx: Forgive yourself. Instead of creating escape fantasies in which you stop the disaster and save lives, instead of berating yourself for your last irritable words to someone who never came home, and instead of feeling guilty, forgive yourself the way you know other people would forgive you if they could. We can only do what we can do at a given moment, we only know what we know, and if we made a mistake, that's what we have to live with. Self-blame stands in the way of acceptance and normal life; by forgiving ourselves, we accept our true limitations.

Rx: Give yourself permission to feel better. It's possible that you may have mixed feelings about allowing yourself to heal. When the pain lets up, it raises distressing questions about how deeply you really cared about the losses of the disaster. Don't worry! To think that all your pain will disappear in a day or a week is one of our great American myths. Sometime during the first four weeks after the disaster, some of the pain should start to let up. It doesn't mean you're insensitive; it means you allowed yourself to feel your feelings fully, have moved through them, and are beginning to come out on the other side. Though everyone moves at a different speed despite the Myth of the Neat Stages, you may make some real progress in the next few weeks.

Rx: Reach out to those who are grieving in the following ways:

- **Allow them to formulate their own alternatives** without overwhelming them with advice or threatening their sense of self-confidence.
- **Do not deny their sorrow and loss.** Reminding them that the person they're grieving for had a good life or died without pain won't help their separation anxiety and may make them feel guilty for thinking of themselves.
- **Don't stay away.** Although they may be withdrawn, upset, or proud, even silent company offers security.
- **Offer social and work activities without pressure.** Don't try to guess what is appropriate for them; everyone handles reengagement differently. Let them know that they're welcome to join life rather than mimic death. It doesn't imply disrespect for their loss when they function as fully as they can.

Chapter Six

The First Six Weeks

In The First Six Weeks that follow a disaster, survival takes on a meaning that goes beyond getting out of harm's immediate way: turbulent emotions have to become more balanced, confused thinking has to become more organized, and physical systems have to replenish and heal. Refocusing on daily life—births, marriages, anniversaries, and even holidays—helps and is normal, natural, human nature. In fact, many people are surprised to find that they can choose to live more flexible lives than they did before the disaster. Consider the way Americans have adapted to security checks at airports; long waits at the entrances to synagogues, churches, and other public places; and even detainments and questionings after the September 11 terrorist attacks. Consider, too, how many chose to make their own changes in their lives. Reports find more people founding new charity organizations, fewer people signing up for plastic surgery, and so many young couples deciding to start families right away that a small baby boom has been declared following the terrorist attacks.

But the gradual return to daily routine is not smooth. Some will frequently and painfully rerun the traumatic experience in their minds in order to digest it. Others will avoid the repetitions to spare themselves pain now but pay the price by slowing their recovery. If anyone tells you they know exactly what you should be feeling right now, don't believe it! Remember the Myth of the Neat Stages? But either way, understanding the process is the best way to ease the progress.

REPETITION

As students, we turn new information into permanent knowledge by reviewing. We digest the new information, associate it with old information, use it in sentences, write about it in essays, read about it, and speak about it. Now we're doing the same thing with the life changes created by the disaster. Whether we're digesting the loss of a pet, a personal illness, a divorce, an economic recession, or a terrorist attack, the process is the same. After The First Six Weeks, we're still involved in retrieving and reviewing the disaster. Expect the following:

Compulsive conversations. You may find yourself asking or being asked the same questions over and over again: "Where were you when it happened?" and "Did you have any personal losses?" and "How are you doing?" The disaster is still being processed. Have patience. Understand that each time the story is told—many different times, maybe in different ways depending on the listener—the verbal repetition will help reduce the shock. Every repeated exposure to the painful memory means more familiarity and adjustment and less of the original emotion, a process called *desensitization*. If listeners extend sympathy, we may also feel somewhat comforted. And if the disaster is a shared experience, comparing experiences and offering sympathy helps move us from private pain back into social interaction again.

Theme dreams. The digesting and desensitizing dialogue will continue on into the night, but this time we will be talking with ourselves. Even in our sleep, the brain tries to make sense of new information and integrate it into permanent memory storage, a process that can take as long as two years!

Some of our dreams may be nightmares, but not necessarily all of them. We may dream about variations on the disaster as it actually was, which may help us deal with our fears or wishes about what might have been. We may incorporate bits and pieces of old disasters from our past, providing ourselves with a reminder of how we dealt with it last time. Or our dreams may involve premonitions of new disasters, warnings, escapes, or rescues, preparing us for the next time if it ever comes.

Flashbacks. If we were seriously traumatized—particularly if we saw death and destruction up close—we may experience flashbacks in which we re-experience the intense emotion we felt during the disaster. Though flashbacks may be frightening because they seem to be beyond our control, they are usually part of the healing process. Going through a flashback is very much like watching a movie the second time. The brain looks for clues, trying to figure out what might have been missed the first time. So instead of feeling that flashbacks happen *to* us, remember their function and get involved in the process. At the very least, taking an active role in flashbacks will help restore some sense of control.

ESCAPES

Not only does the mind review the disaster on many levels until it's integrated, understood, and accepted—and we're desensitized—but since pain is associated with disasters great or small, the mind is simultaneously seeking escape. Some of the ways we do this are harmless or even healthy; others can lead us into more stress.

Fantasy do-overs. If reviewing the disaster as it actually occurred becomes too stressful for us, we sometimes try to escape into fantasy and "shoot the scene again." Like "undoing" fantasies, which were described earlier, we go back to the day of the disaster and think about a more tolerable ending. But this is real life; we can't change the script and reshoot, so we emerge from our "do-over" fantasies to be hit with harsh reality again and again. Furthermore, we've not only increased the number of times we're retraumatized, but every attempt to escape the pain we're feeling by escaping into a fantasy of what "could have," "would have," or "should have" been delays recovery.

Drinking and recreational drugs. Although the danger of reaching for quick fixes like alcohol and recreational drugs was already mentioned in Chapter Five, the risk is as great at six weeks as at four weeks. Alcohol and recreational drugs may give us a break from the hard work of processing the disaster, but ultimately the relief is only temporary. Mind-altering pharmacologicals help us forget for a while, but they don't change the way things happened in reality—and reality is what we must return to once we come down. The more time we spend in this kind of getaway, the more healing time we waste. Not everyone, however, will turn to drugs or alcohol for relief.

Prescription medications. The number of prescriptions that physicians write for tranquilizers and sleeping aids typically increases in The First Six Weeks following a disaster. If they bring us the first few consecutive hours of sleep since the disaster or help us focus on taking care of business or loved ones, they may be worth it. But since some of them can lead to dependence, they're clearly for short-term use. And like other escapes, pharmacological interventions can cover up symptoms that are telling us we need to talk more, listen more, or grieve more. Most doctors recommend re-evaluating the need for medication after two weeks.

To the surprise of many, prescriptions for antidepressants did not increase during the six weeks following the terrorist attacks of September 11, 2001. Those seeking counseling complained of other problems: sadness, yes; anxiety, yes; severe depression, no. Although mood may be "depressed" or energy may be "depressed," true depression will come later, if at all.

MEALS, WHEELS, AND WORK

About one month post-disaster, it's not uncommon to find that our interest in food has returned—not only anxiety eating, comfort eating, and "what-the-heck" eating, but also eating for the pure fun of food. Fast food and real restaurants become a way to venture out again—after all, we have to eat anyway. Cooking and eating together with family, friends, colleagues, or even strangers helps us move back into daily life, which is what we're programmed for and what makes us happiest. And regular meals are one way we can give ourselves the reassurance of knowing what's coming next, which is vital to StressRelief.

About the same time as our interest in meals revives, our interest in wheels may kick back in as well. Earlier, we were in our car as we got back to basics, such as stockpiling food and supplies for the house, picking up children's clothes for the fall, or carpooling. We were in our car, too, when we went to get our quick fixes and small comforts, whether they were cigarettes, a movie, or to help out in the emergency room. But at one month to six weeks, we are more likely to start to use cars for pleasure trips and optional travel as well: a visit to a friend because we're hungering for companionship, or a trip to a wedding or anniversary party that hasn't been canceled. We may even find ourselves buying presents for the car—new mats or a real car wash. These presents are of course for ourselves . . . something to make us feel special, and less guilty than if we were spending on a larger purchase, like a whole new car.

When it comes to work or business life, it may be surprising to see that by the end of The First Six Weeks, daily routines seem to be fully reestablished. We seem to be built for work and love, and we need the reassurance that a regular schedule and paycheck give us. Investors tend to get back to investing, since making choices feels like an antidote to the lost sense of control a disaster brings. And for those who do not have a wide circle of social contacts, work will be a way to re-engage and recover.

THE PHYSICAL FORECAST FOR THE FIRST SIX WEEKS

The term *psychomotor agitation* sounds serious. It's often not. It refers to the toe tapping, leg jiggling, and finger drumming that come with high adrenaline, irritation, or fatigue. But the consequences of psychomotor agitation can be more serious. Waiting in lines may become more difficult now, as may sitting in meetings, taking slow elevators, commuting, and even having conversations. If avoiding these activities makes you feel better, you are more likely to repeat the withdrawal and soon your physical symptoms may lead you to psychological ones, too.

Counter psychomotor agitation with any physical exercise—burn up adrenaline (so it won't drive you) and make yourself physically tired instead of emotionally tired (as a bonus, you'll sleep better).

THE PSYCHOLOGICAL OUTLOOK FOR THE FIRST SIX WEEKS

At the end of six weeks, most of us can expect to feel like recovery has started and shell-shock is beginning to wear off. Instead of bouncing back, however, some find they are retreating. Use this checklist as a guide:

____ Smiles are infrequent, and I don't laugh. I find I don't even smile in situations I used to find amusing, funny, or enjoyable.

____ My senses seem dulled and food tastes flat. My favorite meals no longer tempt me. I eat only to quiet hunger.

____ Sleep is still a problem. I can't fall asleep or stay asleep, or I wake up very early.

____ Sensual activities like a backrub give no pleasure. I seem to be numb.

____ Socializing is difficult. When I'm with friends or family, I feel a million miles away.

If you are experiencing any *one* of these reactions to stress at the end of The First Six Weeks, you are probably emotionally exhausted. This does not necessarily mean you are not recovering. Trying to close down, conserve energy, and reduce emotional demands to prevent further stress is normal; the feeling of depression is most likely temporary and will begin to let up over the next few weeks.

If, on the other hand, you are experiencing *many* of these reactions and your ability to concentrate is so altered that it's hard to function at work, it's time to speak to a family doctor or mental health specialist. If you have ever experienced depression before or were depressed going into the disaster, you are at higher risk of developing a post-traumatic depression and may already know which helping professionals to turn to.

EMOTIONAL CPR FOR THE FIRST SIX WEEKS

The concept of Emotional CPR—choosing thoughts and behaviors to influence your emotions—should be familiar by now. The three "Don'ts" below are especially appropriate for the end of The First Six Weeks.

- **Don't confuse the acute pain and initial anxiety with sadness.** If you think you will always feel this bad, you have not been through a disaster before. The acute pain and anxiety usually let up between six weeks and two months.

The chronic pain and anxiety are usually resolved by two years. But though the pain and anxiety may stop, sadness can, and often does, last forever. This doesn't mean we can't experience joy, love, and excitement. We can, and will. And we will think less often about the trauma. But the sadness when we do think about the disaster may always be there.

- **Don't be afraid to laugh.** Around the six-week mark after a major disaster, we can expect to hear the first few jokes about it. At first they may strike us as tasteless or disrespectful, but they do have a purpose: Laughter is a natural StressRelief mechanism. We are not callous; we are alive. The smaller the disaster, the sooner the jokes will start. And if the disaster was, for example, bank computers accidentally sending huge sums of money into cyberspace, the jokes could start that day since losses were digital, not human. So enjoy the laughter. It releases the body's own stress-reducing biochemicals, and blocks anxiety and fear.
- **Don't stop talking about dreams and flashbacks.** The repetition in dreams and flashbacks helps desensitize us to the disaster. The thoughts and feelings of dreams and flashbacks will be less frightening in the light of day than in the middle of the night when we're alone and waking up in a cold sweat. Furthermore, when we allow ourselves to talk about dreams and flashbacks, we give others around us permission to talk about theirs. We're reassuring them that

their experience is not uncommon and giving them an opportunity to reassure us of the same thing.

The Myth of the Neat Stages is a reminder that suggestions for earlier chapters are still potent for many of us now as well. Here are more:

STRESSRELIEF PRESCRIPTIONS FOR THE FIRST SIX WEEKS

*Rx: **Stick with routines and schedules.*** Familiar patterns are reassuring, particularly to children and the vulnerable elderly. Bedtimes are especially important, because for every hour that our sleep pattern is thrown off, the body needs twenty-four hours to readjust. The early morning light is the most powerful cue for resetting the body's biological clock. So no matter how late we stay up watching newscasts about the disaster and no matter how late we stay up thinking about a personal disaster, our assignment is to get up at the regular time the next morning and get going. If you're tired, go to bed early the following night.

*Rx: **Take one task at a time.*** Before the disaster, you may have been a multitasker and even loved having many balls in the air at once. But now you may be so distracted and processing so much new information that one ball is more than enough to handle. So much of the brain is busy trying to digest the disaster that multi-tasking is likely to lead to errors and failure that increase stress.

Rx: *Pause five times a day.* Just five breaks a day of five minutes each can cut stress symptoms in half, according to Harvard University research. Use the break in any way that turns off your fight-or-flight response: phone a friend; do a crossword puzzle; listen to music; browse a book store; get a backrub; say a prayer; clean your wallet; play with a child; pot a plant; pet a pet; take a walk; or think of yourself as a camera and savor the image of someone being helpful, something of unusual beauty; or whatever pleases the mind's eye.

Rx: *Join a group.* Groups are not only often more effective than most individual psychotherapies for disaster stress, but they also provide an opportunity for making a public statement. Try joining or organizing such a group. Among the community group activities around the country which followed September 11 were:

- Church and school bells ringing in unison
- Candles flickering at every street corner
- Patriotic hymns in karaoke bars
- Special services in houses of worship
- Moments of silence
- Concerts and sing-ins
- College and university chapel services and symposia on issues raised by the disaster

- Prayer vigils
- Poetry readings and music
- Parades of police cars and fire trucks
- A day of reflection in schools featuring readings, art creations, and performances

Rx: Talk to yourself! By now you know that when others remind you that things could be worse, their efforts are not likely to have an affect. But research finds that our mood does lift when we give *ourselves* the same pep talk. So do it! Focus on the positive and remind yourself that there is still much to be thankful for.

Rx: Allow yourself to feel better. During the first month, it was unrealistic to think that we should be feeling no pain. But by the end of The First Six Weeks, the pain usually begins to dissolve—and some people actually feel upset when it does! The lifting of the pain leads to questions about whether we really cared as much as we thought we did and worry that we're not showing proper respect. But the lessening of the pain simply means that nature is doing its work and that we are moving toward StressRelief.

Chapter Seven

The Second Month

During the first few weeks after a disaster, most of us are experiencing similar reactions to the trauma because the built-in fight-or-flight reaction is so powerful and universal. By The Second Month, however, it has become clear that we are experiencing disaster fallout and recovery at different rates. It's more obvious than ever that symptoms can layer themselves on top of other symptoms and that they don't always follow in a preordained order: One person begins to smile again, while a colleague is still irritable; one person is sleeping all night, while a spouse is hypervigilant; and depression descends on some of us and not others.

Although we may recover at different rates and experience different clusters of symptoms, what I call the Sequence of Recovery does seem to be shared by most. That's because the Sequence of Recovery after a disaster reflects our natural, inborn recovery capacities. Healing happens around the clock, even during sleep. Digestion of the disaster continues through conversations, thoughts, and dreams. If losses were deep, we express our pain with sighing and release it with crying. Waking up each morning may still bring pangs as new realizations sink in. Some days are better than the one before, and some are not—but all are evidence that there's been progress in the three phases of the Sequence of Recovery.

THE SEQUENCE OF RECOVERY

The phases that follow are not carved in stone, but most people pass through most of them—how deeply or how long is up to the individual.

Phase 1: Back to basics. By The Second Month, most disaster survivors are well into the first stage, the back-to-basics stage. It probably began within days of the disaster as we began to do whatever was necessary to care for ourselves and others: shopping, cooking, mending, and paying bills. Even now, in The Second Month, taking care of these basics may feel unimportant compared to the disaster, almost sacrilegious: What about the really important things, like collecting disaster-relief funds, mourning the lost, or meditating on life and death? But when a disaster turns entire lives upside down, looking after food, shelter, and other needs helps us survive—it's nature's plan. Getting back to basics is part of getting back to normal, and by The Second Month, we are usually deep in daily life.

Phase 2: Meals and wheels. This phase probably began a few weeks after the disaster. Initially, we ate in order to live; we got into the car because it was the way to get to work, the market, or a memorial service. But soon after the beginning of The Second Month, eating and moving around may once again be about pleasure. Interest in cooking a fine meal, ordering takeout, or inviting people in for dinner may come back. Likewise, our list of driving destinations may expand from the workplace, the store, and the temple or church to the movies, the video rental store, other people's homes, restaurants, and maybe even the highway for no good reason other than a change of scene. Though these may not seem like examples of the survival instinct, they are. An infant who doesn't get enough warm human contact will fail to thrive, and adults are no different. We do best when we care for others—and are cared for in return. In fact, studies show that people with wide social circles live longer than those who have minimal contacts. Reaching out is post-disaster life support.

Phase 3: Quick fixes. This is the phase of the Sequence of Recovery that may need extra attention in The Second Month. By now, some may have tried to ease disaster-related pain with alcohol, drugs, cigarettes, or too much food. Not everyone will turn in this direction—a survey by the American Institute for Cancer Research two months after the September 11 terrorist attacks tells us that only two percent of Americans admit they were drinking more. But since alcohol sales began to rise in this month, those who were drinking more seem to have been drinking a lot more!

THE PHYSICAL FORECAST FOR
THE SECOND MONTH

It is a good time to take inventory of those substances you may be putting in your body to see whether temporary self-medication has become a more permanent bad habit. Start with a reality check. It won't help to read the following, but studies find it does make a difference when you tell *yourself* the following:

- Drugs won't bring back the person we lost.
- Anxiety eating, comfort eating, or "what-the-heck" eating aren't long-term substitutes for the love we miss and may leave us with a weight problem and obesity-related diseases.
- Heavy drinking won't make it easier for us to keep going to work or maintain our health.
- Nicotine in cigarettes won't make us healthier either in the long run, no matter how nostalgic and self-possessed they may make us feel right now.
- Caffeine may ward off fatigue's errors and accidents, but it will also disrupt tonight's sleep so we'll need more caffeine tomorrow.

As you take back control from physical quick fixes, however, freed feelings may rise to the surface. Observe them, understand them, and let them run their course.

THE PSYCHOLOGICAL OUTLOOK FOR
THE SECOND MONTH

By The Second Month, anger may rise to the surface. The first response to an emergency is the release of so much adrenaline that it carries the survivor through the immediate period of rescue, damage, loss, arrangements, and basics. But once the initial fight-or-flight reaction begins to fade, we often find great depths of anger. In fact, *we may go looking for anger to replenish the energy that has drained away.* Anger makes our blood flow, blood pressure increase, and adrenaline levels shoot up. Unfortunately, it also has the potential to set us up to follow angry leaders, whose charisma may lead in the wrong direction. Hate groups often flourish after disasters; in fact, the Southern Poverty Law Center in Montgomery, Alabama, has recently reported a large increase in hate groups after the terrorist attacks. Better, of course, to use anger for good. Make the choice: If the disaster was a national one, direct your anger to patriotism that will motivate hard work for charity groups or military support. If the disaster was more personal, direct your anger to important litigation, rearranged relationships, or personal recovery. We have more control over the direction of our emotional expression than most believe. And taking control brings StressRelief.

DEPRESSION IN THE SECOND MONTH

Immediately following a disaster, most survivors feel anxious; if depression is to come, like anger, it usually doesn't develop until The Second Month. In fact, two months after the terrorist attacks on New York and Washington, seven out of ten Americans said they were having periods of depression, according to a survey from the Pew Research Center for People and the Press in Washington, D.C. This is because by six to eight weeks, the body has spent its supply of the feel-good brain chemical serotonin, depressing the brain center that regulates eating, sleeping, alertness, body temperature, and sexual rhythms. The result may be a feeling of mild depression, a too-large or too-small appetite, too much or too little sexual desire, and trouble falling asleep or staying asleep. If the depression becomes more severe, the pattern will become more clear: Interest in eating, sex, and humor often disappear altogether; hopelessness accompanies the morning, and those Three G's rule the day:

Guilt. Those who survived a disaster when others didn't may feel increased survivor guilt in The Second Month, and the loss of a parent may carry extra guilt about angry words and withheld love. Even getting back to basics may trigger guilt about not dealing with major losses and big emotional issues every minute.

Grieving. In the second month, a tide of powerful grief may come back in and wash away our sense of coping. Then, bumping into people who didn't know about the loss forces us to review it again and compounds the grief. Our heart becomes heavy, and the dawn is dark.

Grim predictions. For some disaster survivors, trying to picture a future worth living is still an exercise in frustration because the loss still feels too great. For others, a negative past is all there is to project into the future. For still others, the disaster is just the first in a series of traumas to come.

People with previous psychiatric problems may feel the negative effects of severe stress even more about now. So as time goes on, if panic attacks, phobias, other anxiety conditions, the Three G's, or uncontrollable emotions increase, it's time to make an appointment with a physician or counselor.

EMOTIONAL CPR FOR THE SECOND MONTH

Two months after any disaster—great or small, personal or national—routines have usually been re-established, though powerful emotions may still be playing themselves out. It's the time to see whether any emotional quick fixes, like drinking, smoking, overeating, or drug use, have become part of the daily routine. The Emotional CPR tips that follow can help you resist these emotional crutches. Since our feelings follow from our actions, take action now.

Prepare to quit smoking. There are many programs available to help those who would like to quit smoking, or any destructive behavior, but you can get a head start with these do-it-yourself basics. To prepare yourself for quitting:

- Make a list of reasons to quit (kids, health, budget).
- List the immediate benefits (more stamina, less coughing, a sweeter-smelling house) and post it where you can see it many times a day.
- Make it public. Announce your intentions to those close to you. This signals commitment.
- Turn your goal into numbers, so it can be measured or charted—like the number of hours without a cigarette, number of cigarettes smoked, or number of dollars saved.
- Create a plan. Expect to feel nervous, anxious, and hungry—so . . .
- Choose the starting week carefully! Try for a routine-filled week, but don't put the start date off if there are none.
- Think of ways to keep your hands busy (yoga, sculpture, worry beads).
- Think of ways to keep your mouth busy (singing, carrot sticks, chewing gum).
- Think of ways to keep your brain busy (brisk walks, a new health-club membership, books on tape).
- Go to places where smoking is not allowed (libraries, movies, restaurants).

■ Now, choose to start, and reward yourself for very small successes—points, stars, or a CD—*not* food!

Examine your drinking behavior. The biggest obstacle to kicking an alcohol habit is denial: denying the problem and denying the need for outside help. To assess the problem, confront yourself and ask if drinking has interfered with your job, friendships, or family life for at least a month. If the answer is "yes," the diagnosis is alcohol abuse. If you have also built up a tolerance, need a drink to function adequately, or suffer from withdrawal when you try to stop, the diagnosis is alcohol dependence. Whether you drink every night, drink heavily only on weekends, or go on "benders" from time to time, the problem is still alcoholism, and alcohol is running your life—and you're not! Though some people can get control of their drinking on their own, outside help may make it much easier to stick with sobriety when stress or disaster hits again.

Kick your drug habit. If you feel insecure without a supply of any psychotropic (mood-altering) drug, prescription or not, if you lie or feel guilty about your drug use, miss social occasions because of it, are spending too much time and money on it, have developed a tolerance to it, or sneak away from work or family to use it, you need help. As with alcohol, kicking a drug habit may go more smoothly with outside help. But you can try this Emotional CPR first:

- Identify the emotions from which you're trying to escape—often loneliness, boredom, anger, or stress—and address them directly and constructively.
- Try going drug-free one day a week, then two, then more, until you're drug-free every day.
- Reward yourself with praise and pampering. Using drugs less often means having more money!
- Fill your free time with enjoyable activities, preferably in public places with people who don't use drugs.

Stop overeating. According to research done about ninety days after September 11, people eat more after a disaster. There are many reasons besides hunger: as a distraction from annoyance, worry, or loneliness; to delay doing something unpleasant; to fill up when empty of love, affection, or warmth; or to comfort with favorite foods, to return to the good old days with old-fashioned or home-cooked food. If overeating is a personal problem, take a moment to look inside and see if you might be eating for emotional reasons. Once feelings are acknowledged and greeted, the desire to eat too much may fade; the following tricks can take you the rest of the way:

- Schedule all snacks and meals and enjoy them.
- Eat snacks and meals at the table only. The calories from on-the-run snacking add up.
- Go low-fat and low-calorie, so you never feel deprived.

- Drink lots of water since thirst can be confused for hunger.
- Exercise to control hunger—not to build it.

Rx: Seek out the real fixes. If unhealthy quick fixes such as smoking, alcohol, drugs, and food have taken center stage in your life, it's time to put something else in the spotlight! After confronting the emotions, which are usually the main reason quick fixes tempt us, fill your life with *real* fixes that work, don't do damage, and support forward motion:

- Work it out with exercise.
- Get your hands dirty—gardening, carpentry, doing repairs.
- Take a walk with a child or dog and remind yourself what it's like to feel enthusiastic.
- Try a new skill and then share a project with a friend.
- Pamper yourself for a full hour.
- Clean out your wallet, drawer, or closet; it restores a sense of control.
- Watch cartoons if they make you smile.
- Give StressRelief—get StressRelief. Do volunteer work.
- Create a journal and review it regularly. Become an observer of your own behavior. Watch with humor.

- Add some music to your life: listen, play, or sing.
- Pray or meditate.

Rx: Try cinema therapy. After the September 11 attacks, restaurant revenue went down, but Americans apparently spent more money at the movies than at any time since World War II. In fact, moviegoers paid nearly $100 million to see *Harry Potter and the Sorcerer's Stone* in its first weekend two months after the tragedy. It's possible that the film would have been a huge hit without the tragedies, but it didn't hurt that it had for its theme a mysterious, alien, evil force conquered by children who are kind, brave, persistent, and pure of heart. Because of this universal theme, it's also possible that parents nobly taking their children to see Harry Potter got something out of the movie, too.

Movies are more than just entertainment. In times of transition or uncertainty, scary images from our real lives are replaced by movie images we know are make-believe. We can lose ourselves for a few hours, and there are no announcers cutting in with bad news. If the movie is the first in a series, it promises a future we can look forward to. At the movie house we come together for a safe emotional experience with other people, hear the laughter, and share the tears. Movies can make us feel better—cinema therapy—and during tough times, here are the categories that relieve stress best:

- **Comfort movies.** These films are so familiar we can recite almost every line; because of this predictability, the brain goes off alert and relaxes. Try *Grease* (if you were alive in the seventies, you know every song!) or *The Godfather* (the guys in my family know every word!).

- **Classic war movies.** These remind us that we've been through difficult times before and came out on top. Try *Casablanca* (tough guy becomes patriotic and noble) or *Mutiny on the Bounty*.

- **Family movies.** The movies in this group make us feel cozy and reminiscent. Classics are *The Sound of Music* (a war movie and true story about a family that survives World War II and ends up in the United States) and *It's a Wonderful Life* (perhaps one of the most uplifting movies of all time, one that reminds us of the value of community).

- **Movies with humor.** Laughter is nature's antidote to stress . . . so use it! Recent favorites, according to box office reports, are *There's Something About Mary* (painfully funny, as one reviewer put it) and *Home Alone* (kids find this one gives real StressRelief).

Chapter Eight

The Third Month

The three-month point is the 90/90 point: By that I mean 90 days after a disaster, about 90 percent of us have resumed daily life. For many, there's a welcome drop in hyperventilation, hypervigilance, and hyperactivity; appetite, natural sleep patterns, interest in sex, and sense of humor are on their way back. On some days, life feels almost like it did before the event.

Around ninety days, however, some may be also hit with delayed reactions. Sometimes it's because they came to tragedies or emergencies pre-sensitized because of past traumas in their personal life, so the fallout goes on and on. Sometimes it's because they tried to blunt the pain with drugs, alcohol, instant intimacy, or food, postponing the shock of realization. More often, it's because they waited until they caught their breath before letting in the pain. Delayed pain is duller pain, and many chose dealing with duller emotional pain for longer periods of time over feeling earlier sharper pain for shorter periods. For them, the impact will dissipate more slowly, but it's a trade they will take—or must take.

As with most disaster-related symptoms, these delayed reactions are usually normal responses to an abnormal situation. But though they're normal, they're more than normally stressful because they no longer serve the survival function for which nature designed them. Symptoms may also cause special trouble if they're not obvious and don't seem directly linked to the trauma. By The Third Month, the disaster is no longer in our thoughts every minute; we want to be doing better and assume we are doing better. This is why we may not consciously connect the symptoms to the trauma. Men may attribute exhaustion or depression to the flu or a cold. Women may write off headaches, emotionality, easy tears, or difficulty concentrating as hormonal. Maybe they are, in fact, related to colds, flus, or hormones, but quite possibly they're not. It's wise to be suspicious of symptoms that appear as if by magic ninety days after a trauma.

THE PHYSICAL FORECAST FOR THE THIRD MONTH

The long-term physical stress symptoms of a disaster are very much like the long-term physical stress symptoms of running a marathon. While the runner is running, levels of the stress hormone cortisol rise to ease the working of the joints and keep down inflammation; once the cortisol level drops after the race, the runner is more likely to have a flare-up of allergies, skin problems, and some kinds of arthritis. And like distance runners who are advised to be extremely careful about exposing themselves to viruses and bacteria for a few days after they run because the stress of the race wears down the immune system, people under traumatic stress are also more prone to colds and infections. Other body systems may also have been so busy coping with the emergency and preparing for injury and illness that they're worn down and vulnerable to a long list of flare-ups. They can appear any time during the months following the trauma but are especially likely to emerge at around ninety days, when physical resources often reach rock bottom. The most common ones are:

- Headaches
- Neck aches
- Backaches
- Asthma
- Allergies
- Constipation
- Diarrhea
- Stomach "knots" or "butterflies"
- Nausea
- Heartburn
- Peptic ulcers
- Irritable bowel syndrome
- Ulcerative colitis
- Rheumatoid arthritis
- Hyperventilation
- Dizziness

- Muscle spasms
- Esophageal spasms (swallowing difficulties)
- Panic attacks and cold sweats
- Urinary frequency
- Insomnia
- Memory impairment
- Chronic fatigue
- High blood pressure
- Cardiac arrhythmia
- Chest pains
- Myocardial infarction (heart attack)

Some of the symptoms on this list are mere inconveniences, but others, like heart attacks, can be life-threatening. When worrisome physical symptoms like these emerge, passively waiting for the stress level to come down may not be enough to preserve health. Taking active steps toward StressRelief is crucial.

THE PSYCHOLOGICAL OUTLOOK FOR THE THIRD MONTH

While many of us feel by The Third Month that our psychological resiliency surprises us more every day, our psychological resources can be as depleted as physical ones. When that happens, the pep talks that boosted our spirits in the first three months may not work as well anymore. The adrenaline that provided energy for working on a rescue team or rebuilding a life after a death dwindles and the small amount that does flow isn't enough to give us a lift. The psychic energy spent in the last ninety days on learning that we're strong and that there's life after trauma, the work we did surviving the nightmares and flashbacks and becoming more desensitized to the trauma, and the hypervigilance, hyperventilation, and hyperactivity—all may have played themselves out, and nothing has taken their place. It may seem as if we're going through the motions of living, allowing apathy to run our life—and we couldn't care less.

This apathy is not the same as depression. Often, appetite and sleep remain normal, and serious feelings of hopelessness or worthlessness are not in the picture. What is present is the simple desire to do nothing much. The mind feels finally, totally exhausted. Energy-yielding adrenaline and cortisol levels have disappeared, and so has the support system we relied on: Cheerleaders, boosters, counselors, and good friends probably assume all is well by now. They include us in their plans less often and don't extend their nurturing as readily as before. We're usually not taking good care of ourselves anymore, either, because we think that after three months. it's inappropriate to keep ourselves on our own critical care list . . . we think it's time to check ourselves out and go home. But The Third Month may be too soon for many of us.

People who are physically and emotionally depleted can't imagine that they will ever feel different than they do today. They look into the future and see a haze. It was easier when, during

The First Week, seeing our way to the end of the day was as much future-casting as we could manage or expect of ourselves. During The First Month, the sight line stretched as far as a week ahead. By the end of three months, forward planning can reach a month into the future and possibly far beyond that. But for those who have had a great loss, the future may seem very large and very empty. Even though the initial shock was months in the past, the psychological renovations and rebuilding that will make the future more comfortable are still incomplete. Though it may not be a conscious thought, an uncertain future can very much affect decisions made in the present.

EMOTIONAL CPR FOR THE THIRD MONTH

At ninety days, the waves of acute emotional pain may have eased off and heavyhearted sighing may have stopped, but the healing still isn't over. The grief, the guilt, and the grim predictions may take as long as six months to ease, maybe longer. And remember that it takes two years before the brain doesn't have to remind itself on waking of the great loss. At ninety days, the body, mind, and spirit need as much attention as ever—maybe even more if symptoms are intense and have gone on so long that they interfere with work, relationships, and other aspects of daily life.

Since our emotions can be led by our actions and thoughts, hang around optimists for Emotional CPR. If the future seems empty and apathy is the ruling non-emotion, choose your com-

panions wisely! Make a conscious effort to surround yourself
with optimism and relaxation and avoid a lot of face-to-face time
with people who are "down." This doesn't mean you should suddenly shed all stressed friends. But attitudes are contagious, and
ninety days may mark a serious low point. It's healthful to try to
balance the stressed friends with an equal-sized group of people
who are action-oriented.

STRESSRELIEF PRESCRIPTIONS FOR THE THIRD MONTH

Rx: Behave "as if." When getting back to full function is difficult, remember to once again behave "as if":

- When you feel anxious, behave "as if" you felt more calm.
  Soon your brain and emotions will follow your actions.
- When you're feeling apathetic, act "as if" you want to get
  up and take care of the yard work or project. Since you have
  probably had a better attitude about the yard work or project in the past, the old feeling may come back in the environment where the accomplishment is to take place.
- When you're feeling asocial, like crawling into a cave by
  yourself and hibernating for years, force yourself to get out
  and do some socializing. It will distract you and probably

spark a new series of invitations and friendships. They will, in turn, pull you out of the cave and into the sunlight.

Rx: Celebrate. After ninety days, people are looking for reasons to celebrate. Weddings, charity functions, and patriotic events are all legitimate and may be attended with relief and pleasure from the knowledge that it is still possible to do something so normal. In fact, any holidays that fall around the ninety-day mark are usually celebrated with gusto, even by those of us who are still grieving. And we're sometimes even ready to think about taking a vacation again.

Rx: Connect. By ninety days there's more face-to-face contact than before, including lunch appointments, dinner plans, and holiday family gatherings. Movies seem more inviting and sports, both those played and those watched, become more interesting again. And most of us have rediscovered our interest in sex. This is probably a built-in step in recovery, since satisfying sex increases endorphins, which are natural mood elevators and painkillers; serotonin, a calm-down, feel-good brain chemical; dopamine, which suppresses appetite; and prolactin, which promotes sleep.

Rx: See your doctor for medical concerns. If chronic digestive problems develop, if an existing problem such as irritable bowel syndrome (IBS), migraine headaches, or allergies suddenly gets much worse, if the menstrual cycle becomes erratic, or if any unexplained symptoms appear, see a doctor. He or she may not only be able to help prevent chronic problems but can make suggestions about psychological or spiritual counseling if needed.

Rx: Hypnotize yourself. Don't abandon the StressRelief exercises that appeared in earlier chapters of this book simply because it's been ninety days since the disaster and time is up! You can and should continue to do the StressRelief Breathing and Progressive Muscle Relaxation mentioned in Chapter One. Let your body know it's time to relax with this classic autohypnosis exercise from Stanley Fisher, Ph.D., author of *Discovering the Power of Self-Hypnosis: The Simple, Natural Mind-Body Approach to Change and Healing*:

1. Sit comfortably in a chair facing a wall about eight feet away. Pick a spot or an object on the wall about a foot above your sitting eye level. This is your focal point.
2. Look at your focal point and begin counting backward from 100, one number for each breath you exhale.
3. As you count and continue to concentrate on your focal point, imagine yourself floating, floating down, down through the chair, very relaxed.
4. As you stare at the focal point, you will find that your eyelids feel heavier and begin to blink. When this happens, just let your eyes slowly close.

5. While your eyes are closed, continue to count backward, one number for each time you exhale. As you count, imagine how it would feel to be as limp as a rag doll, totally relaxed and floating in a safe, comfortable space. This is your space.

6. As that safe, comfortable feeling flows over you, stop counting and just float.

7. If any disturbing thought enters your space, just let it flow out again; continue to feel safe and relaxed.

8. To come out of autohypnosis, either let yourself drift off to sleep, or count to three and exit using the following steps. At one, let yourself get ready; at two, take a deep breath and hold it for a few seconds; at three, exhale and open your eyes slowly. As you open your eyes, continue to hold on to that relaxed, comfortable feeling.

Rx: Talk, talk, talk. If daily life has lost its rhythm, if your personality seems changed rather than just shaken up, or if physical or psychological symptoms are not abating—start talking! Remember that the one in ten relief workers who suffer from Post-Traumatic Stress Disorder (PTSD) after a disaster are generally offered group crisis intervention. Family physicians and religious leaders are good sources for support groups. Research finds groups even more effective than individual therapists for this kind of post-traumatic reaction. Trauma victims need people to listen, respond, and sympathize . . . and the more listeners in the group, the more response and sympathy are available. In a group, ideas tend to flow and concepts of all kinds are voiced . . . and usually found to be more common, benign, and more manageable than they had seemed. In fact, someone in the group may be a perfect match for our own experience and feelings. Consider that just about any group, even one not led by a professional counselor, can be full of "therapists" who can help you—and the time and expense of group therapy is usually less than that of individual therapy. Family physicians and religious leaders are good sources for support groups, but if symptoms don't go away, the hours and cost of individual therapy may be well worth it instead.

Rx: Listen, listen, listen. If you're the one who's trying to help a disaster survivor, whether it's at ninety days or ninety minutes, let them talk. Don't block what they're saying, don't pacify it, and don't reject it. Now, as much earlier, listen hard; then repeat back what you've heard (known as active listening). This lets them know you were really listening carefully and gives them a chance to hear their own feelings again. If you feel awkward about any part of this process, just remember that most survivors are grateful to see your face, hear your voice, and have you near. To give them needed control, encourage them to make plans without doing it for them. To give them needed motivation, let them know when you'll be checking in with them next.

*Rx: **Be open to the new view.*** After ninety days, we may look back on the event and suddenly find that it somehow looks different, a phenomenon called "reframing." What seemed to us to be a very personal event last month may suddenly take on political significance this month. We may suddenly find that we have learned beneficial lessons from the trauma or may have a more realistic view about how uncommon this kind of disaster is.

*Rx: **Take breaks—they still help.*** At ninety days, we may begin to feel confident we can stop "wasting time" taking breaks, but our minds and bodies can still use them, especially if our support system is paying less attention to us and the relief workers have gone home. By ninety days, emotional exhaustion creates a double susceptibility to depression and worry, and we're much more likely to avoid them if we parent ourselves now. Defend your right to meditate; review diet and exercise; set aside time for sleep and friends.

*Rx: **Smile.*** Because you can probably go minutes or even hours without thinking of the trauma now, you may finally be able to smile again. Humor becomes enjoyable instead of offensive— and you may even find yourself pursuing it, since happiness floods the body with endorphins, which can take the edge off of both physical and emotional pain. When you're standing at the gift wrap line or supermarket check-out counter and time is passing, smile instead of grumbling. Attitudes are contagious! If

103

laughter has been elusive in the last three months, you may find it again during the next three. Laughter turns off adrenaline, increases pain threshold, and helps create a feeling of community—the best kind of StressRelief to share.

THE UNCERTAINTY INVENTORY

Most disasters don't end on Day One. Earthquakes have aftershocks, deaths have implications, and terrorism is an ongoing threat—all of which create uncertainty. Though at 90 days after a disaster about 90 percent of us are back to routines, we may still feel the stress of living with uncertainty as we worry, watch, and wait. Measure your own uncertainty stress level by giving yourself one point for each of the following symptoms, which are at least sometimes true for you:

___ I hop from one task to the next to the next, often finishing none of them.

___ I feel confused sometimes about which way to go when getting off an elevator, or I forget where I am when driving down the road.

___ I jump when the telephone rings or a horn honks.

___ I drum my fingers or twirl my hair nervously.

___ Bad weather can really ruin my day.

___ Long check-in lines at the airport or department store make me feel like I'm about to explode, and sometimes I do.

___ Traffic jams and crowds make me feel hemmed in.

___ A stuck elevator makes me feel panicky, and I feel like I have to escape.

___ It takes me forever to fall asleep at night.

___ I wake up many times during the night.

___ At night I have the same bad dreams over and over again.

___ I'm tired when I wake up, tired after my coffee break, tired in the afternoon, and tired all day.

___ When my partner approaches me for sex I'm receptive, but I'm never the initiator.

___ Things that other people think are funny I think are stupid or silly, and I hardly ever laugh.

___ I cry much more than I used to.

___ Singing patriotic songs, listening to music from my parents' youth, or hearing "our song" chokes me up.

Now add up your points. If you have just *one point*, you are stressed by uncertainty. If you have *three or more points*, you are very stressed by uncertainty. Here are some suggestions for making areas of uncertainty more stable and predictable:

1. **Stick to routines.** Load up your life with predictability; your adrenaline level will drop and so will the symptoms.

2. **Take one task at a time.** For months after a disaster, many of us will be too distracted to multitask. Take it slow and restore your feeling of control.

3. **Plan ahead.** Expect the unexpected, and leave lots of extra time for lines and traffic. If you don't, you'll be pumping up your adrenaline levels even more.

4. **Get angry.** In recent decades we've seen the terrorist attacks of September 11, acts of cruelty by a madman in the Oklahoma City bombing, tragic school shootings at Columbine, air disasters, and assassinations. If you feel anxiety due to the resulting uncertainty, let moral outrage create a warrior! Get active within your community to ensure public awareness. Press for safer schools. Write letters to Congress people. Use up your adrenaline because this kind of healthy, life-preserving, and goal-directed anger is incompatible with fear and cancels anxiety.

Chapter Nine

The Sixth Month

Morning shock begins to quiet down about six months after a disaster. Since the brain has begun to understand on all levels that something has changed permanently, the shock of remembering every morning when we wake up, and the pounding heart that goes with it, are much less common now; we awaken with knowledge instead. For better or worse, morning shock may be replaced by morning sadness. The startle response begins to return to the resting state, and the body is no longer on constant alert. Concentration is returning, restful sleep is now possible, and a good meal or good sex may be once again enjoyable, even sought after. For some there's a new enthusiasm about the coming day— for others, just a new day. Either way, by six months most have reentered their daily world, and being out and about encourages contact with other people and fosters forward motion. Recovery is usually well underway.

Disaster upon Disaster

As with all healing, however, some recuperations are more complicated than others. A disaster recovery may proceed without complications if the disaster ended cleanly—but disasters rarely do. Sometimes, disasters have aftershocks: An earthquake may lead to a move or the eventual loss of a job; an accident may lead to a long jury trial. In the case of terrorism, fear of new attacks may cause new trauma. And dabbling in quick fixes like alcohol or drugs may not only delay healing but create new mini-disasters of their own.

Then the cascade of stress hormones will continue to flow. But the stress system that activates during a disaster is basically a short-term system, meant to prime us for survival in the hours following a disaster. It's true that some time-release endocrine-system hormones are also released to keep the brain and body primed for lifesaving action over the subsequent days and weeks, but when disaster follows disaster and adrenaline is still flowing six months after the original event, the stage is not only set for fight or flight, but also for great wear and tear.

The Physical Forecast for The Sixth Month

If the body has been on constant alert for six months and has not had a chance to rest, the effects of chronic stress usually start to show. Constant anxiety often means more missed heartbeats, rapid beats, or the occasional pounding sensation—after all, the heart is a muscle, not a machine, and muscles tire and spasm. Breathing patterns also change under stress, becoming more rapid the rate can as much as double and more shallow, like panting. Short term, these changes help us fight or take flight. After The Sixth Month, they can leave our mouth and nose dry and our chest in pain as the diaphragm muscles cramp from working so hard in the struggle for breath. If the fast, shallow panting goes on and on, we may have "panic attacks" from hyperventilation. If the stress hormones continue to flood our nervous system, we may end up with cold feet and hands, a sallow or pale complexion, migraine headaches, or high blood pressure as our blood flow is shifted to large skeletal muscles and decreases to the gastrointestinal tract and to the skin. Add slower and desynchronized (irregular) contractions of the digestive system and the vasoconstriction of gastric glands under stress, and we may develop upset stomachs, diarrhea, or constipation. And since stress hormones can suppress immunity, we may develop one of many kinds of infection, inflammation, or even cancer.

Exhaustion at this time may have to do with the fact that the endocrine glands are still signaling the well-intentioned release of extra energy-giving sugars into the bloodstream. But because the body is on high alert, it may produce more than enough insulin to break down these sugars for use—and blood sugar levels drop to such a low level that we feel shaky and tired, a condition called *hypoglycemia.* The urge is to quick-fix the problem with sweets, cola, coffee, or cigarettes; but then the body responds with even more insulin, and the low-blood-sugar cycle continues (try complex carbs or a dairy snack instead). Finally, long-term stress may find its way to pre-existing physical weaknesses (see Chapter Four) and aggravate them. The heart, stomach, intestines, lungs, and skin are likely trouble spots, causing serious conditions such as heart attack, ulcers, ulcerative colitis, asthma, and more. Be alert for physical stress symptoms, be in contact with your physician if a problem develops, and consistently follow the StressRelief Prescriptions appropriate for you.

THE PSYCHOLOGICAL OUTLOOK
FOR THE SIXTH MONTH

By six months post-disaster, our individual differences in circumstances and coping ability are even more dramatically obvious than before. Those of us who brought to the disaster a strong support system and a history of sensible eating, frequent exercise, and general good health usually have very few chronic stress symptoms now. If, however, the most recent disaster is just one in a string, if there's been the loss of a parent, loss of a job, an out-of-sequence death (say, of a child—the parent always expects to go first), or personal illness before or since the disaster, we may find ourselves at six months in that smaller group of people who haven't yet re-engaged in daily life. The inventory of Emotionally-Toxic Shock symptoms may be bulging: Depression (which sometimes is just beginning at The Sixth Month) and the

Three G's (guilt, grief, grim predictions) may be too much with us. Unusual amounts of fatigue, insomnia, back pain, and moodiness may color each day. Gorging, bingeing, compulsive eating or dieting, difficulty swallowing, dramatic gain or loss of appetite, and dramatic gain or loss of weight may be stealing our energy and good nature. And finally, the addictions—alcohol, drugs, smoking—may have us in their grip. Our psychological outlook at The Sixth Month, then, has a lot to do with our psychological history. StressRelief Prescriptions take this into account. So should we all.

Gender also accounts for many post-disaster differences.

GENDER-SPECIFIC
RESPONSES FOR WOMEN

Women are at risk not only for all of the general symptoms mentioned so far, but also for a specific group of ailments that affect women only. Stress can easily tip the delicate balance of hormones that direct female functions of all kinds. The result can be:

Increased premenstrual syndrome (PMS). PMS is already somewhat of a trial for nine of ten women, and the stress of a disaster can make its headaches, hot flashes, anxiety, nervousness, bloating, fatigue, irritability, depression, breast tenderness, temperature changes, food cravings, thirst, acne, allergies, and other symptoms even worse. According to gynecologist Sharon B. Diamond, M.D., of Mount Sinai Medical College in New York,

111

stress influences the brain's hypothalamus gland, which in turn activates the pituitary and thus the ovaries, which are the source of the progesterone and estrogen involved in PMS. Stress can easily and efficiently upset the delicate hormonal interplay and aggravate PMS symptoms. It's also likely that PMS makes stress worse, says Peter J. Schmidt, M.D., of the National Institute of Mental Health. His example: If someone hits you on the arm, you feel it. If someone hits you on a sore arm, you *really* feel it. He found that women in the premenstrual phase felt stressed by life events that didn't bother them at other times of the month. Imagine what happens when PMS combines with a life event that *does* bother us at other times of the month—such as a disaster!

Pregnancy problems. Stress is known to cause amenorrhea (absence of menstruation), conserving blood and iron that a woman may need in the face of stress. We also know that high levels of stress can in rare cases cause irregular ovulation and fallopian tube spasm, making conception more difficult, according to the American Society for Reproductive Medicine. Mother Nature may be protecting her own: Pregnancy not only means health concerns for the developing fetus, but also may mean morning sickness, weight gain, and lack of exercise. Then add withdrawal from alcohol, nicotine, and some medications, worries about impending medical and hospital bills, concerns about wage-earning changes, and fears about lost time and freedom— not an ideal state of mind for a couple during times of trauma.

Although a time of terror or trauma may not seem ideal for a pregnancy, many actually choose pregnancy anyway during these times in order to reaffirm their hope in the future! In fact, after the September 11 attacks, a seize-the-day mentality came over many men and women of baby-making age: You may remember that at least one dating service experienced a mini-boom in business, the media reported numerous stories of long-engaged couples deciding to finally get married, and Steven Brody, M.D., says Alvarado Hospital Medical Center in San Diego received about 25 percent more calls than usual from men and women wanting information on overcoming infertility. People were seeking security and looking to rebuild, and what better place to start than with a family?

Sexual dysfunction. Although stress and its quick fixes often interfere with a man's ability to become aroused and get an erection, a woman often has a less obvious sexual reaction to stress: anorgasm (lack of orgasm). She may become aroused, but an orgasm becomes more difficult to achieve since she is distractible and vigilant. It is not uncommon for vaginismus (painful intercourse caused by spasms of the pubococcygeus muscles surrounding the entrance to the vagina) and inhibited sexual arousal (formerly known as frigidity) to also appear, or reappear, about now. As the tensions of the trauma let up, expect these sexual symptoms to let up, too. If they don't, or if they preceded the disaster, ask your family physician for a referral to a specialist. Or contact the American Association for Sex Educators, Counselors, and Therapists in Washington, D.C., for a few names and then interview each before making a decision.

Post-partum depression. Depending on which study you read, between 20 and 65 percent of childbearing women report maternity blues. Since postpartum (after-the-birth) depression rarely begins before the third day after delivery, it seems clear that hormonal changes are more involved than psychological changes, but stress can also play an important role. Giving birth is already an enormous emotional event; having a baby under stressful circumstances is even more so. Is bringing a child into the world a good idea? How joyful can the occasion be if the father was lost in the disaster? The mother's first days at home with the baby can be a blend of joy, wonder, and aching loneliness. If the newborn is a boy, he may remind her of her loss—another mixed blessing.

Menopause melancholia. The end of a woman's fertility is not the negative life event it was once considered to be—many women see it as new freedom from the possibility of pregnancy—so menopause and disaster are not a guaranteed bad match. However, the insomnia and hot flashes of menopause may combine with the insomnia, nightmares, and early wakings of the disaster aftermath to make for some less-than-restful nights.

More female factors. Under stress, women also report more anorexia, bulimia, anxiety attacks, and depression than men. All of these stress-related conditions in turn cause stress on the body that may be long term and beyond control. For example, when women who are already anorexic or bulimic become flooded with adrenaline during a trauma, they are often more vulnerable to other disaster-related ailments than women who have normal eating patterns. And women who are already having anxiety attacks and depression before a disaster are even more prone after the disaster. The sooner that any ailment—physical or emotional—is identified as disaster-related or disaster-aggravated, the sooner its negative affects can be reversed.

GENDER-SPECIFIC RESPONSES FOR MEN

As for the mainly male disaster responses, there are many. We know that, in general, men tend to respond to stress differently than women. Young men often react to stress so nonverbally and act so quickly that both seem to be part of one response. They can stay focused on high-arousal situations intently and for long periods, and may be less aware of low-level pain sensations than women. They may join a disaster rescue team, for example, and work at their task for hours without a break. They may also focus only on their immediate task and postpone focusing on the long-term consequences of a disaster until they begin to unfold. As with the female body, however, the male body has some target areas—and the stakes are sometimes even higher for men than women, including not only disorders, diseases, and dysfunctions, but also death.

The cardiovascular system is where most of the action takes place. Cardiovascular disorders include disorders of the heart (cardio) and the blood vessels (vascular). For men, heart disease becomes the leading cause of death by approximately age forty, whereas for women this isn't the case until around age seventy (most likely because androgens, the male sex hormones, seem to increase blood cholesterol, while estrogens, the female sex hormones, seem to decrease it). Of the many cardiovascular diseases, disorders, and dysfunctions, four are strongly associated with long-term stress in men: hypertension, atherosclerosis, heart attack, and heart failure. In fact, decades of research on the relationship between stress and cardiovascular disease have convinced the American Heart Association that stress is a secondary cardiovascular disease risk factor, interacting with the primary controllable risk factors of hypertension (high blood pressure), high serum cholesterol, diabetes, smoking, lack of exercise, and obesity.

Hypertension. Hypertension refers to chronic high blood pressure. Blood pressure rises if the heart rate increases or the arterial blood vessels constrict, which they do under stress. Short term, this adjustment can be useful; long term, it can be perilous. Heart contractions in the average man occur about seventy times per minute—that's about 40 million times a year—and pump more than 2,000 gallons of blood a day. During exercise, sexual arousal, or stress, the number of heart contractions per minute can double, doubling the strain on the heart muscle and the arteries. This type of increase in blood pressure creates no danger if it's infrequent and transient, but it may be a major danger if a cardiovascular problem already exists—or if stress goes on and on during disaster-fallout.

Atherosclerosis. In atherosclerosis, fatty deposits build up on the inner lining of the arteries, raising blood pressure and reducing blood flow to the heart muscle and this happens even faster in the presence of prolonged high blood pressure and stress. Soon the walls of the arteries are less elastic and less able to cushion the higher systolic pressures generated by the heart, and a vicious cycle has started. The longer the stress goes on, the longer the increase in blood pressure—and the greater the amount of fatty deposits, especially cholesterol, which is used throughout the body for mending membranes. As the cholesterol continues to coat the inside of the arteries, blood pressure continues to increase, and so on. Although we get many of the ingredients for manufacturing cholesterol from the foods we eat, such as egg yolks, dairy products, and animal fats, most of the cholesterol circulating in our bloodstream is probably manufactured in our own liver. Once it is deposited on arterial walls, cholesterol or a blood clot can block an artery entirely or break off and block a smaller, more peripheral vessel that leads to the brain.

Heart failure. The heart may enlarge to do the work it has to do, but its blood supply may not increase proportionately. Soon it will tire like any other muscle and spasm painfully (angina pectoris) because it's not getting enough oxygen, or maybe even fail.

Heart attack (myocardial infarction). A second danger is that high blood pressure will burst an artery or push a blood clot or mass of foreign material into a small vessel. If this deprives tissue of blood, it will die (infarct). When the tissue affected is brain tissue, the condition is called a cerebrovascular accident or *stroke*. When the tissue affected is heart muscle, the condition is a heart attack or *myocardial* (heart muscle) *infarction.*

Cardiovascular events are not the only ones that touch more men. Among the other mainly male ailments and ills and ailments:

Alcoholism. Male alcoholics outnumber female alcoholics by about three to one in the United States. This means men are particularly vulnerable to alcohol abuse, alcohol dependency, or using alcohol as self-medication after a disaster. Short term, alcohol can be a sedative, disinhibitor, muscle relaxer, and soother of survivor guilt. Long term, it's likely to disturb sleep, affect the intestines, impair motor coordination, and slow down StressRelief because it's an escape from dealing with the real disaster fallout.

Sexual dysfunction. A disaster is not as likely to directly affect a man's sexual function as his quick fixes are! Alcohol, for starters, may make take away inhibitions, but it may also interfere with a man's ability to get or maintain an erection. Marijuana and cocaine can decrease desire; in addition, marijuana and amphetamines can contribute to erectile dysfunction. Mood-management drugs such as fluoxetine (Prozac), paroxetine (Paxil), sertaline (Zoloft), and many heart and blood pressure drugs can lower libido and/or cause erectile dysfunction. However, as with women, a disaster may also be a sexual stimulus.

Ulcers. Stress may increase stomach acidity and tax the immune system, eroding the stomach or intestinal wall and allowing bacterial infections to cause painful ulcers, possible bleeding, and potential death. And under stress, people trying to self-medicate may also drink more alcohol, smoke more cigarettes, and gulp down more coffee and tea, which can worsen any ulcers already there. Statistics indicate that men are somewhat more prone to ulcers than women are, though the gap is not as large as once thought.

Other male factors. On top of these risks, men are more apt to minimize or deny their pain than women, and that usually means they are seeking treatment much later in the disease process. They may also be so unaware of physical problems that they wait until symptoms are impossible to ignore. According to the Men's Health Network, a Washington, D.C.-based advocacy group, men are two times less likely to visit a physician than are women.

EMOTIONAL CPR FOR
THE SIXTH MONTH

Even though many disruptive emotions have leveled off by The Sixth Month, your mind and behavior can still take the lead in fine-tuning feelings. All of the Emotional CPR (Cognitive/Psychological Resuscitation) strategies from previous months still apply. Check the list below and customize the collection of StressRelief Prescriptions for yourself, since no two people have exactly the same needs.

As we have said before, healing often requires behaving "as if" you are interested in daily life again—but what we didn't say before is that behaving "as if" can shape not only your own future but that of others, which is a great gift you can give. At three months, for example, you may have felt less than interested in food or sex. Going through the motions "as if" you were interested may have led to more enjoyment and less stress; now, by six months, you may be ready to take the initiative and bring other people along. Likewise, at three months, smiles may have returned; now, at six months, laughter that everyone can share may be coming back. Acting "as if" can make it so because stress hormones respond to the brain's call for action; stop calling for action and the body can finally find rest as adrenaline levels drop below the radar.

StressRelief Prescriptions for The Sixth Month

Rx: Prioritize. At six months, it's time to make sure some life-preserving business has been taken care of.

1. **Check your physical health.** At six months, we're not as physically overloaded as at the peak of the emergency, but it's actually now that wear and tear are most likely to become evident. Ailments at this time may be disaster-related.
2. **Check your emotional health.** If the Three G's (guilt, grief, or grim predictions) or depression are the emotion of the day—every day—see a counselor or a physician for a referral.
3. **Check loved ones' physical health.** Are they ailing bodily? Are they refusing invitations for reasons of illness or physical discomfort? Do what you can to help and heal.
4. **Check loved ones' emotional health.** Has anyone you know dropped out of social interactions? Are they depressed? Again, see that they get help.

Rx: Get physical exercise. If you feel tired, lethargic, isolated, withdrawn, sleepless, or sexless, physical exercise can help get the body back on track. Exercise pumps up circulation, releases endorphins (the body's natural painkillers), and is an opportunity

121

to get out and be with other people, even if it's just to run side by side on a treadmill. Morning exercise and grabbing daylight on cloudy and snowy days (take a daytime walk even if it's just during lunch) will help reset your body's daily clock.

Rx: Pause. Even at The Sixth Month, breaks from stress hormones are still necessary . . . maybe more so than ever, since for many people recovery at six months is in a deep physical and emotional valley. Revive the habits of StressRelief Breathing (Chapter One), Progressive Muscle Relaxation (Chapter One), and autohypnosis (Chapter Eight).

Rx: Play. What movies came out in the last six months? Which sports teams are ahead, what music groups have had hits, and what shows are big on Broadway or on TV? What games did your child, niece, or nephew get for a recent birthday, and do the new swings at the playground need a test drive? If you don't know, it's time to find out. Young people provide special opportunities for fun. But putting the play back in your life can actually be more than fun—it's healthful. An Israeli study showed that young people who closely monitored news reports about a disaster were more likely to suffer from Post-Traumatic Stress Disorder than those who distracted themselves with games or caring for others.

Rx: Set the alarm. Even if you feel a disaster has wrecked your schedule completely, even if all you want to do is eat and sleep, push yourself to get up at the same time every morning, on the early side if possible. Remember, the body needs early morning light to reset its biological clock each day. When you wake up tired, plan to go to bed earlier tonight rather than sleeping in now.

Rx: Announce your intentions. Broadcast the news that you're about to dump addictions and break bad habits. Tell the world you're going to quit smoking, stop using drugs, and not drink so much anymore. If you can't keep yourself honest, let the rest of the world help. No excuses! Get tough now, since problems tend to grow, not dwindle. A specialist can guide you though cognitive therapy, behavioral therapy, group therapy, or medication if necessary. (See Chapter Seven, The Second Month, for specifics on escaping the grip of substance problems.)

Rx: Head off PMS. Now that premenstrual syndrome is no longer considered to be a mental health issue, physicians and health care professionals have become open to the idea that it may be correctable or at least modifiable—and if you are a woman, doing so is wise when disaster stress is threatening to drag you down. Among the prescriptions that physicians may recommend for some women are antiprostaglandins, tranquilizers, selective serotonin-reuptake inhibitors, calcium, progesterone, vitamin B6, diuretics, and bromocriptine (for breast tenderness). Home remedies include cutting back on salt intake to reduce water retention (don't overdo this in the summer) and aerobic exercise for thirty minutes a day, which may help fight depression and flushes extra fluid out of the body. Many women find that minor changes in diet make a big difference; eliminating alcohol and caffeine, for example, can reduce outbursts and irritability. An increase in carbohydrates may help to increase brain serotonin, which in turn may reduce depression, tension, anger, confusion, sadness, and fatigue, and increase alertness and calmness. Maybe this is why some of us crave carbohydrates premenstrually; we may be trying to self-medicate with potatoes, bread, pasta, cake, and candy! (Not the best way to go.) Instead, try six small meals rather than three big ones. This reduces hunger and prevents bingeing on sweets.

Rx: Head off menopause symptoms. If a disaster makes menopause symptoms more unbearable than they would ordinarily be, estrogen/progesterone replacement therapy may relieve the discomfort (and may also slow osteoporosis). Options for women who are not candidates for hormone replacement therapy because of a history of breast cancer, blood clots, or other disorders include topical solutions such as water-soluble jellies that relieve vaginal dryness. Consult your physician for more information.

Rx: Head off heart disease. If your cholesterol count climbs and your blood flow dwindles, worrying about future heart attacks can add stress to stress, and maybe even increase heart-disease risk. Fortunately, there are a number of things people can do improve their risk profile. Among them:

- Change eating habits to reduce cholesterol intake and also of animal (saturated) fats, which seem to encourage the liver to produce cholesterol precursors. Cutting fat also cuts calories and leads to weight loss.
- Increase exercise to "use up" the noradrenaline, epinephrine, and fatty acids that pour into the bloodstream during stress. Exercise also cuts calories and leads to weight loss.
- Consult a physician about taking medication to lower blood pressure or increase tranquility.
- Get diabetes under control.

Chapter Ten

The One-Year Anniversary

Fifty-two weeks, 365 days, a whole year between the disaster and today…they make a comforting cushion against the pain, and a promise that survival is real. Laughing is probably easier now, sleeping may no longer require pharmacological assistance, food has probably gone beyond sustenance to become a reason to gather with friends again, and sex may once again be a pleasure. This is not to say that life is necessarily "normal." One year after the Oklahoma City bombing, for example, a Gallup poll found stress was running almost two times higher in Oklahoma City than in neighboring cities, the rate of dreams or nightmares about the bombing was 2.39 times higher, and people there were drinking 2.5 times more than Indianapolis residents. At one year, the disaster is far from forgotten—it may never be forgotten—but it's often no longer in our minds every waking and sleeping minute. Things seem to be moving forward—toward "normal." But then….

The One-Year Anniversary of the disaster may take you by surprise. The distance that separated the present from the past disaster may seem to vanish as memories and feelings come flooding back with surprising force and vividness. Some survivors talk about feeling as if the disaster were suddenly "just yesterday" again. It's called the *Anniversary Reaction.*

THE ANNIVERSARY REACTION

Not everyone will have to deal with an Anniversary Reaction, and those who do deal with it will not all experience it to the same degree—once again, it's the Myth of the Neat Stages. But the one element everyone shares, of course, is the time when the Anniversary Reaction occurs, and in addition, the reaction does have several fairly consistent elements:

Cues. Whether or not the date of the disaster is in conscious memory, something about the name of the month, the smell of the air, the weather conditions, comments from other people, or media coverage triggers memories and feelings. The reaction can begin before, during, or after the anniversary depending on awareness of its impending arrival, the length of the original event, and our response to it.

Replay. Because the experience seems so real, the days surrounding the anniversary of the disaster may feel very much like the days surrounding the disaster itself. Depression, anxiety, guilt, anger, insomnia, nightmares, intrusive thoughts, and other symptoms may get worse, and that can be discouraging to those who thought they were getting better. It's possible that survivors will not only re-experience their old emotions but actually suffer new injuries as they go through the re-experience under new circumstances—it's called *retraumatization*. Some residents of Littleton, Colorado, the site of the Columbine school shootings, said they felt retraumatized by the observances of the anniversary, even the well-intentioned ones, such as memorial events and sympathetic news coverage.

Surprise. One of the most difficult aspects of the Anniversary Reaction to deal with is the surprise. For the first eleven months after the disaster, most survivors feel they are steadily returning to normal. They take care of business during the "back to basics" phase, interest in food and outreach returns during the "meals and wheels" stage, and though a few detours into "quick fixes" such as drugs, alcohol, smoking, or too much food may be explored, they're usually resolved. All of these normal reactions to an abnormal situation seem to be leading toward life as it once was, or something reasonably close. In this context, an Anniversary Reaction can hit unexpectedly hard and be very discouraging. It helps to know that the Anniversary Reaction may come, and it helps to be ready.

Reframing. The farther we stand from a painting, the fewer details we see. So it is with a disaster as seen from the one-year perspective. Looking back, the details may be fading by The One Year Anniversary, and the bold outlines becoming more vivid. After a war, an act of terrorism, or an earthquake, for example, the nation remembers the heights of heroism, the loss of life, and the cost of rebuilding, but not the daily disruption and clean-up. So, too, after a personal loss, we may remember great acts of kindness or love or generosity or foolishness, but, again, details may begin to fade. It's important not to feel guilty if this process begins—it's natural and leaves us with an image we can bear to look at every anniversary.

Revising. Have you noticed that nations reinterpret history to fit their current policies? Acts of war are remembered as acts of peacekeeping, civil unrest recalled as resistance, and public protest redefined as patriotism. We do the same, so that our past will fit neatly into our present. If we've gone on to start a family or business or changed a career, we have to see the past trauma as a catalyst for the current "good"—or we may feel too guilty about having moved on so well. If there's no current good and our loss cannot be repaired, the disaster may become a "warning" or a "lesson," in retrospect, to reduce our bitterness.

PREDICTING YOUR ONE-YEAR OUTCOME

Because we all enter traumatic events with different histories, strengths, and vulnerabilities, we all come out differently, too.

And some of us may find that we have not healed as well or moved as far as we would have liked by The One-Year Anniversary of the disaster. If that is true for you, it may be for one or more of the following reasons:

1. **Lack of control** during or after the disaster. An accident, trauma, or loss that threatens our sense of control over events will have a more lasting negative effect than one that doesn't. For example, passengers in car accidents are eight times more likely to develop phobic travel anxiety than those who were drivers in car accidents.

2. **Persistent health problems** before or after the disaster. Chronic pain disrupts sleeping, eating, sexual pleasure, concentration, and physical exercise. Is it any wonder that persistent health problems will interfere with post-traumatic healing as well as everyday life and ambitions?

3. **Constant rethinking and rumination** after the disaster. Negative interpretations of the disaster and intrusive memories (flashbacks) are strong predictors of the one-year outcome, increasing the probability of someone suffering anxiety or Post-Traumatic Stress Disorder four to seven times. It may be that some victims overgeneralize the danger that follows their disaster. It may be that they see the fallout to be life-threatening when it isn't, or more frightening than it should be.

4. **Financial loss or legal difficulties** during or after the disaster. When we're "hit in the pocketbook" by a disaster, the

economic bruises can last longer than physical bruises. We may feel we did not "take care of business," anticipate the disaster, and protect our assets. If our self-worth is tied up with our financial success, there may be more guilt, anxiety, and depression after one year than after one month! And if financial trouble or litigation continues, the continuing reminder of the disaster will most likely interfere with a natural tendency toward symptom resolution.

The point of this review is that early recognition and prediction of chronic problems can help you arrive at your first anniversary after a disaster with as much support and intervention as you need. If you think your recovery is not all it could be, perhaps you now have a better idea about why that is so. Sometimes the problem can be "fixed," and sometimes not. Either way, knowledge is power.

BENEFITING FROM THE ANNIVERSARY REACTION

During anniversaries we automatically recall and review. The process seems to be built-in and hard-wired. What can be the benefit of returning to the emotional state of a year ago? What possible use is re-experiencing pain and loss? How can reliving a disaster be anything but disastrous itself?

The answer is that remembering marks our passage and our healing. The commemorative events reassure us that we're in this together and making it. All societies through time have created memorials—particularly first-year anniversaries. They are attempts, say sociologists, to end the feelings of uncertainty and uneasiness that we've passed through for the last year, and represent a pledge to move on. The anniversary is an opportunity to look at the disaster from a new point of view—one year out—and reframe what happened using that information. If you've wondered about your strength and resilience, this may be the time to acknowledge how far you've come. If depression, anxiety, guilt, anger, insomnia, nightmares, intrusive thoughts, and other symptoms revive around the one-year point, they're asking for attention. Give it to them. If you've started to sweat the small stuff again, this may be your opportunity to regain your perspective.

PERFECTING YOUR PERSPECTIVE

In the days following a disaster, victims may be literally unable to write down a list of life's positives. A disaster can overrule the tiniest happy thought. But by The One Year Anniversary, some moments of joy should be filtering through and strength should be returning . . . often in the form of a new perspective: "I'll never sweat the small stuff again." My research in The Stress Program at Mount Sinai Medical Center in New York has found that within forty-eight hours, promises like these often are forgotten and perspective has slipped back to where it was before the promise—but not always.

In my family, perspective is permanent because my mother is a 10-, 20-, 30-, 40-, *and* 50-year survivor of cancer. Each time she was faced with the ordeal of surgery and the process of recovery, the entire family reviewed priorities. And at every one-year anniversary of her surgery, we would do the same. Now we always hold on to health and happiness over small worries. Although no disaster is a good disaster, a major disaster will most likely alter our perspective permanently. I predict, for example, that the terrorist attacks of September 11 will give us a focal point for perspective alignment that won't be likely to fade within forty-eight hours. We will use our experience of the disaster and the days and the months that follow to remind us every anniversary for the rest of our lives that our national security, freedom, health, and safety are priorities—and traffic jams and slow elevators are not.

The good news is that the discomfort of the anniversary reaction generally lasts only a few days, then recedes again—perhaps for another year. If strong emotions seem to return more frequently than once a year, it's possible that the anniversary reaction is occurring monthly, weekly, daily, or randomly. One young woman who had lost her father on a Saturday continued to feel distressed on weekends until she identified weekend activities as triggers for her memories. If you can identify your triggers and cues, you can turn down the volume of your anniversary reactions much more quickly, since they will no longer take you by surprise.

EMOTIONAL CPR FOR
THE ONE-YEAR ANNIVERSARY

One year after a disaster may be an especially challenging time for disaster survivors because emotions may be at a higher pitch than in past months. Emotional CPR may be especially useful now. So plan for the anniversary instead of hoping it will slip by.

Although it's natural to dread the first anniversary of a disaster great or small, to want to ignore it, planning for it allows you to take control and guide your emotions. Without a commemorative service or ritual as a focus, calls and words of sympathy may spread over weeks. If the tragedy was shared by a community or a nation, the memorials may stretch through too many excruciating days and nights. Make sure to schedule some very private time to grieve. Anniversaries can be too big to bear unless there is planning. Paying your respects is healthy. Paying the price of re-immersion is not.

STRESSRELIEF PRESCRIPTIONS FOR
THE ONE-YEAR ANNIVERSARY

Rx: Accept your feelings. When a disaster was a national experience, media rebroadcasts around The One-Year Anniversary may stir up old hurts we thought were gone. Comments from well-meaning friends will bring back that out-of-control feeling . . .

and our pain. Expect it all, let the feelings flow, and the tears, too, if they come. Expressing emotions is always the quickest way to move past them, and it's especially true with the Anniversary Reaction.

Rx: *Take an inventory.* Disaster victims may say that it's been almost a year and they're still not over it, that they're still suffering, that they're still mourning, and that not a day goes by that they don't think about it. But when a therapist, counselor, or family member looks at certain specifics (see the list below), it turns out that the victim has made progress without realizing it. If you feel stalled—or if an Anniversary Reaction has set you back—place a check mark by the statements that are true for you now and see how far you've come:

___ StressRelief exercises have calmed me since the disaster. Prayer or meditation have helped me feel better since the disaster.

___ I've taken part in ceremonies, observances, or other group activities since the disaster.

___ Substance problems or addictions had a grip on me— until I got a grip on them.

___ Fears and phobias were running my life—until I got help and demystified them.

___ Physical problems threatened to overwhelm me—until I saw a doctor, made a plan, or took action.

___ I've stopped blaming myself for what happened.

___ I sleep much better than I did right after the disaster.

___ My dreams and flashbacks don't seem strange to me now.

___ I talk about dreams and flashbacks with others.

___ Grief and pain are still with me, but they're not as acute or constant as they were before.

___ I've accepted invitations to go places and do things since the disaster.

___ I've extended invitations to friends and acquaintances since the disaster.

___ I smile much more than I did at first.

___ I've caught myself laughing in the past year.

___ I actually had some fun in the last year.

Scoring: If you marked *any* of the statements in the checklist above, you've taken at least one big step toward recovery. Scan the unchecked statements for ideas about what steps to take next.

Rx: Don't confuse the anniversary reaction with depression or seasonal blahs. It's easy to assume that feeling down or "off" as The One Year Anniversary approaches is really spring hay fever, fall allergies, the start of school, waning winter light (a winter blues condition called Seasonal Affective Disorder), or just plain depression. But if negative feelings seem to come and go on a regular basis, make a note of the month, day, or condition of their onset. Does it relate in some way to the month, day, or condition of a disaster in the past? If so, you now know why the antihistamines or light therapy didn't work. Now you can begin to treat the symptoms with the prescriptions at the end of every chapter in this book—and get real StressRelief.

Rx: Find a support group or see your therapist more often.
The support group for survivors of a major Virginia flood in November 1985 sponsored a covered-dish supper in a church a few days before the anniversary of the flood. On the anniversary evening, the group also encouraged residents to put lighted candles in their front windows, which served, in the words of one survivor, as "a memorial to those who died in the flood, as a tribute to those who worked in flood relief, and as a symbol for the undying spirit of those who have survived the flood." The large community response was heartwarming and healing. If the Anniversary Reaction hits so hard it flattens you, you may need group support too, or outside help. Though the reaction usually fades within days, those days can be unbearable for some. If the reaction goes on and on, a therapist can help you make it through this year and prepare for next year.

Rx: Distract yourself. Around the time of the anniversary, remember that you have choices: You don't have to watch every TV special on the disaster, keep the radio on 24/7, or attend every memorial service. Choose one or two meaningful observances, and then find something else to do. Movies work well, many say, because they replace the thoughts and sounds in our heads with fresh dialogue, music, and new images. (See "Try cinema therapy" in Chapter Seven.)

HOLIDAYS: A SPECIAL KIND OF ANNIVERSARY

Holidays are already difficult anyway—we're busy, we're entertaining, we're stretched to the limit financially, and in the case of winter holidays, we may be struggling with the desire to go into hibernation!—but holidays can be especially difficult for people who are dealing with and healing from a disaster. A holiday is not an anniversary of a disaster, but it can be a year-ly window into how life used to be before everything changed. The view can very disorienting and dislocating: Traditions of the past become meaningless, a place at the table is empty, and there's the potential to "overcelebrate" with too much food, too much alcohol, too much spending, and too much smoking. Raw emotions can mean easy arguments and crying. Here are some guidelines for surviving holidays as they interact and combine with disaster—and preventing them from becoming mini-disasters themselves:

1. **Plan time with family or friends who are nurturing, welcoming, and happy.** Spend as little face time as possible with those who are not.

2. **Create one or two new traditions to mark this holiday as different.** That way you'll be less apt to compare it to the past.

3. **Keep it low key.** A quiet, meaningful celebration is what many disaster survivors want and need.

4. **Be realistic.** Don't expect a picture-perfect holiday celebration this year. It was never picture-perfect in the past—why should it be now? Gift-wrap lines won't be faster, airport security screening won't disappear, and Uncle Henry is not going to be friendlier this year. Focus on what you can control, like good food, music, and company.

5. **Converse with constraints.** Discuss, don't debate; communicate to be heard, not to win; share information and facts, not opinions and angry words; focus on the future with hope and try not to look back with nostalgia.

6. **Don't compare your holidays to anyone else's, and stop thinking that yours are not good enough.** That is mental cruelty and probably inaccurate anyway.

7. **Avoid overeating, overdrinking, oversmoking, and overspending.** Getting a grip will give a needed sense of control.

8. **Pause often.** Time may be tight, but we all need a break

from adrenaline. Massages and yoga classes make great gifts—for others and also for yourself.

9. **Attend religious or spiritual services.** The familiarity, rhythmic chanting, gathering of congregations, and meditation time are all stress relievers.

10. **Remember that celebrating holidays is natural.** Holidays are life-focused, good for children, and a way of bonding with family and community.

11. **Get professional help if the holidays are more burden than blessing.** Watch for these trouble signs:

   - Loss of appetite
   - Increased isolation
   - Difficulty falling asleep or staying asleep
   - Agitated or slowed-down behavior
   - Constant fatigue
   - Sadness
   - Difficulty thinking or concentrating

And On Into the Future

It's natural for disaster pain to slowly recede as the years intercede. Thinking about the disaster, talking about it, and revisiting it all help with the process of desensitization and integration. However, in a handful of cases—about one in twenty-five Americans—the pain evolves into chronic Post-Traumatic Stress Disorder (PTSD). Symptoms of PTSD usually begin about three months after the traumatic event, but sometimes they don't show up for years. Hardly anyone has all of these symptoms, but a diagnosis of PTSD is appropriate when there is evidence of at least one of the "re-experiencing" symptoms below, three of the "avoidance" behaviors, and two instances of "heightened arousal":

Re-experiencing: Flashbacks, nightmares, intrusive memories, and uncomfortable feelings or physical stress reactions when exposed to emotions, sensations, places, or people that bring the trauma to mind.

Avoidance: Trying to avoid sensations, places, or people that bring the trauma to mind; numbed emotions; inability to remember part or all of the trauma; loss of interest in everyday activities; limited activities; a sense of futility; expectation of early death.

Heightened arousal: Irritability, angry outbursts, troubled sleep, poor concentration, an exaggerated startle response, and hypervigilance.

Rx: Remind yourself that Anniversary Reactions are normal and temporary—and may even be part of your healing. After the anniversary, you'll probably pick up where you left off, and you may even be stronger.

If the trauma is sexual assault or childhood abuse, it's possible that major depression, social phobia, generalized anxiety, or a panic attack will also appear.

PTSD symptoms are particularly likely to appear during anniversaries of the disaster—or when the proper cues are in place. A young man who was in a traumatic accident at age twelve, for example, had Anniversary Reactions until he was twenty-six (that's as far as psychiatrists followed him). In a separate study, two World War II veterans suddenly developed Post-Traumatic Stress Disorder symptoms in 1995—triggered by media coverage that commemorated the fiftieth anniversary of the end of the war!

If you suspect you are suffering from PTSD or know you have severe Anniversary Reactions, add the following Stress Relief prescriptions to those from earlier chapters:

Rx: Inform your family and friends about the way you react. If you were blindsided by crying, hostility, depression, flashbacks, or similar phenomena the last time an anniversary rolled around, it will help to be prepared next time. That includes telling loved ones what might be going on in your mind so they'll understand—and treat you with compassion.

Rx: Get away. If being in a certain place at a certain time triggers memories, arrange to be in a different place on the next anniversary. Removing yourself physically can separate you from many of the cues that will trigger an uncomfortable reaction. The young man described above who had Anniversary Reactions was free of them when he was not in his home town.

Rx: Get professional help. It's normal to feel sad, anxious, scattered, and sleepless after a traumatic event—but not for more than about a month and not to such a degree that your life is totally derailed. PTSD symptoms can persist for years if they go untreated and can place the sufferer in a worsening spiral of negative emotions and consequences, such as depression, drug abuse, alcohol abuse, eating disorders, and divorce. It's important to see a physician, psychologist, or psychiatrist if you suspect you have PTSD. Antidepressants, tranquilizers, desensitization therapy, cognitive behavior therapy, and stress management training can all help to turn PTSD symptoms around. A list of resources is provided at the end of this book.

Chapter Eleven

How to Help the Children

Every parent and adult hopes to protect children from all the bad things that happen in the world. But now more than ever, young people are exposed to events beyond adult control.

By the time children are five or six years old, they're reading headlines and hearing news alerts on television. Children today see more than thirty dead bodies a week on television news programs, many more in movies, and an average of thirty acts of violence in cartoons in a given half hour. By the time they're twelve years old, children have typically been witness to more than 100,000 acts of violence on TV. This exposure, though second hand, should not be minimized. As I've mentioned before, after a study of more than 1,000 school children, researchers at Stanford University found that real-life violence seen on television news programs may have just as powerful an affect on young emotions as an actual terrifying incident. Were children affected by news footage of terrorists flying into the World Trade Center and the Pentagon? Of the Columbine killings? Of the Oklahoma City bombing? Of course. In fact, 63 percent of children, according to one national survey, say they worry that they might die young. Then there are the disasters that may affect our children directly: natural disasters like hurricanes, earthquakes, droughts, tornadoes, floods, and fires, which can take their home; manmade disasters like a war that takes a family member, street violence that affects their neighborhood, terrorist attacks that disrupt their daily life and threaten their sense of security, and car accidents that kill a pet or friend; and family disasters like illness, poverty, abuse, divorce, and death.

How can we help our children get through any disaster and its aftermath, and maybe even emerge the stronger for it? The first vital step is to learn what *children* consider a disaster—which is often very different from what adults consider a disaster. The second is to learn how to spot the symptoms of children's stress—which often differs from the adult version. The third and most difficult step is to learn to help children deal with disaster—which, again, may be very different from how adults deal with disaster. Of course, understanding, support, reassurance, and lots of affection will be part of that, but children today need something else, something more. Read on.

CHILD-SIZE STRESS

If you want to know what children consider a disaster, ask them. I did. For my book *KidStress,* I surveyed close to 1,000 children under thirteen years of age and asked what made them sad and mad and scared. Their answers astounded me! They were not the answers that parents and I had expected—like friends not liking them, other children making fun of them, being punished, or failing at something. The actual answers children gave were so very different from those predicted that we must rethink some assumptions about children's view of disasters. They were less upset by personal and social setbacks than by the loss of loved ones and by the pain of others—the same kinds of events and losses that we adults find most upsetting! They said they get angry about inequality, human cruelty, and disloyal friends. They get scared when their parents fight or they have to be alone, but they also worry about water safety, pollution, and nuclear war—almost four times more than they worry about their personal safety. And loss, illness, or death of a family member (or pet) lead the children's list of disasters. Read some of their responses, and remember that most of the children polled are only between nine and twelve years old:

"I get sad when…"

- Somebody dies or somebody gets their feelings hurt.
- I think about my cat that died.
- A pet or animal gets sick or hurt!
- Someone I love is sick.
- My sister goes away to her school.
- My parents go away on trips without me.
- People get killed.

So many children are so sensitive to loss and the sadness that death brings that we can't just brush these traumas off with reassuring platitudes like "the victims are in heaven now." Once children are about eight years old, they're not likely to forget a disaster, and if it leads to the death of a parent, friend, or close relative, they'll be trying to cope with the single most life-changing stress experience for a child. Other events that can bring trauma to a child's life include:

- **Parents' divorce.** More children see psychologists and psychiatrists for divorce and its aftermath than for any other reason.
- **Natural disaster such as a fire, flood, or hurricane or human disaster such as a terrorist attack or war.** Events like these make children feel frighteningly out of control of their lives.
- **Financial strains in the family.** To the surprise of many parents, children are usually aware of financial stresses in a household. Not only may a child have to forgo clothes, toys, trips, programs, and technological equipment that other children can afford, but tensions usually rise between parents as well.
- **A parent's physical or mental illness.** Children know they need adult help and are traumatized when depression, alcoholism, or other physical or mental problems distance parents physically or emotionally.

- **Absence of a parent.** Most children have separation anxiety when a parent leaves and worry that they won't come back—particularly if it's a trip to the hospital.

The vital task of adults, when children face a trauma, is to cut the trauma down to a child's size, to make it understandable in simple terms and make it manageable day to day. *Children have their own inborn StressRelief capacities!* Very young children may comfort themselves by rocking or sucking their thumb. Preschoolers may act out their fears during play or let out their sadness during make-believe. Older children may ask questions over and over until they've finally begun to process the disaster, may withdraw to conserve their strength, and may daydream about better times. All are normal reactions to abnormal situations. *But children can use these capacities only if they are not overwhelmed.* The adults around a traumatized child must maintain routines so the child has *predictability* and spend time with the child so the child has *reliability.* As much as possible, children should be told what's coming next, and new situations, people, and schedules should be previewed!

SIGNS OF STRESS

Children may not have the words to tell us about their reactions after a disaster . . . but they find other ways:

The Physical Forecast

One way they tell us about their stress is with their bodies. The message they're sending is as clear as if they had used words. If they're confused, their heads throb in an effort to make sense out of the confusion. If their gut is wrenched with fear, their stomach hurts. If scenes on television make their blood run cold, they will shiver and shake. A more complete list of physical symptoms:

- Stomachaches, "butterflies," or "knots"
- Headaches
- Shivering, cold hands, pale cheeks
- Sweating, damp palms, dry mouth
- Dizziness, lightheadedness
- Frequent colds
- Nausea and/or vomiting
- Allergy flare-ups

The Psychological Outlook

When it comes to behavioral symptoms, what we think we see may not be what is really there. Sulking or sudden shyness may really be withdrawal due to trauma. Poor school performance may really be excessive distraction or daydreaming to escape the memories of a disaster. Watch for signs like the following (from the National Institute of Mental Health).

FIVE AND YOUNGER

Although they don't really understand loss and death yet, children five years old and younger feel the disruption in their household during and after a disaster and react to changes in the level of attention they receive. Look for:

- Clinging and fear of separation from parents
- Crying or whimpering
- Unusual screaming
- Immobility or aimless movement
- Trembling or frightened facial expressions
- Regressive behaviors such as bedwetting, thumb sucking, and fear of darkness

SIX TO ELEVEN YEARS OLD

Children in this age span will ask questions about a disaster and how it will affect them or may repeat information they heard on television or from friends, but true logic is not fully developed, and their fears and concerns may be exaggerated or even irrational. They still need a lot of clarification and reassurance. Look for:

- Withdrawal
- Disruptive behavior, outbursts of anger, and fighting with siblings

- Trouble paying attention
- Nightmares and trouble sleeping or sleeping long and heavily (somnambulistic withdrawal)
- Refusal to attend school
- Depression, numbness, and apathy
- Regressive behaviors such as baby talk or interest in stuffed toys or an old blanket

TWELVE TO SEVENTEEN
YEARS OLD

Preteens and teens talk a good game and sound very knowledgeable, but they are still children and have a hard time understanding anything that they have not personally experienced. In fantasy, life can always return to the ways things were before the disaster. Watch for:

- Flashbacks and nightmares
- Numbness
- Avoidance of reminders of the trauma
- Substance abuse
- Problems with peers
- Antisocial behavior and isolation
- Depression, guilt, and suicidal thoughts
- School avoidance and academic problems

CHILD-TO-CHILD DIFFERENCES

Why does one child react strongly to a disaster while another seems to bounce back? Researchers studying identical twins raised apart find that a large part of our reaction to disaster is inherited, our "nature." If one twin tends to be nervous, jumpy, easily irritated, and highly sensitive to trauma, an identical twin tends to be similar, even if raised in a different family. Likewise, if one twin is resilient and willing to see change as a challenge, the identical twin also tends to be like that.

But a child's "nurture" plays two important roles in stress reactions, too. First, adults act as models for children. Younger children especially tend to take emotional cues from the adults in their lives. If they see anxiety, they feel anxiety. If they see calmness, they copy the calmness. Adults' behavior is the pattern they use to learn survival and adult behavior. Second, adults act as a *source* of stress or a *remedy* for stress for children. Even a child with a calm temperament will be stressed if a parent is always highly stressed.

Children may also vary in their ability to deal with stress during different times of their childhood. The twos are terrible enough without extra stress! The teen in the middle of a hormonal hurricane may not be as flexible as one whose rapid growth has finally slowed down. And as with adults, a child may change how he or she reacts, depending on what else is going on in his or her life.

TEENS AND DISASTER STRESS

The teen years are a time when your son or daughter may want to stop being a child but is likely to also fear the responsibilities of growing up. During this time your child might become old enough to drive, vote, and join the military, but not enough of an adult to understand the extent of the danger in the world—so the risk of traffic accidents, drug abuse, and unplanned pregnancy is higher in these years than at any other time in your offspring's life. The emotions teens feel are typically intense, and if they are sad, fearful, angry, or humiliated, they cannot believe they will ever feel better—so the rates of depression and suicide are high in this age group. Then there are the raging hormones and an array of personal crises: self-image disasters, sexual disasters, dating disasters, school disasters, and family disasters. An external disaster can come as a very rude awakening.

To help both your teen and yourself cope, remember that adolescence is a time when both boys and girls start to feel a very strong need to appear, act, and be mature and create a new, adult identity that is separate from yours—but they may not yet have all the skills they need to do so! If teens show an over-the-top stress reaction, it's because they're vulnerable not only to childhood stress responses but also to many of the adult ones, too!

EMOTIONAL CPR FOR CHILDREN

Throughout this book, Emotional CPR has been a tool for adults to use in order to fine-tune their stress response to be more manageable. Emotional CPR works for children, too. The focus will be to increase their sense of security during and after a disaster, because children have *no real sense of control* over their environment. When a disaster hits, they feel their helplessness even more. They're completely in the hands of their family and the other adults around them. The common sense, love, and awareness of these grown-ups makes all the difference between a child feeling protected from the world and a child feeling vulnerable instead. Don't let a child get lost in the emotional fallout of a disaster. Children need to see us taking a break from worrying, taking time to ask questions, and taking time for ourselves. Children will not catch their breath until we do. Don't save your StressRelief Prescriptions for the middle of the night when the children are in bed.

STRESSRELIEF PRESCRIPTIONS FOR CHILDREN

Rx: Child-size the disaster. Explain the disaster in the simplest, most reassuring, terms you can. Let them know how they are being protected. Find some activities to "make things better": Draw pictures as gifts for the bereaved, make food for those in shelters, and so forth. You don't have to explain every detail about the disaster to your child. It may be more than they want to know or need to know, and it may make the stress much worse. And it's not a good idea for them to see disaster images again and again on television. If they are very young, they will think that it has happened many times.

Rx: But don't shield them. You may be tempted to have a moratorium on the news or unplug the TV, but if the children in your life are school-age, they'll find out anyway.

Rx: Ask lots of questions. Have a family discussion in which everyone (including you) is encouraged to say how he or she feels. To get the conversation started, you can ask, "What do you think happened?" or "If you were the President, what would you do?" Listen to all answers and repeat them back to show you heard every word. Children may then qualify or change their statements, which means you've provoked thoughtfulness. When they ask the same question over and over, smile . . . and know that this is their way of digesting tough information. Be on the lookout for physical signs of stress in your children, who don't have the words to express their new feelings of fear: stomachaches, headaches, too much eating or not enough, nightmares, and distractibility.

Rx: Understand that they don't understand. Children can comprehend only experiences they have had themselves. A six-year-old who has never had a relative pass away may think that disaster victims are only sleeping. Even teens may not think logically, fantasizing, for example, that a deceased parent will somehow be back.

Rx: Remind children of the "chain of love." A disaster can stir up fears of losing a parent for the first time, and the experience can leave a child feeling small and alone. One of the best antidotes (for adults, too) is what I call the "the chain of love": "If anything happens to Mommy, Daddy is right here to take care of you. If anything happens to Daddy, Grandma and Grandpa love you and will take care of you. If anything happens to Grandma and Grandpa, Aunt Gretchen loves you and will take care of you. If anything happens to Aunt Gretchen, Mommy's best friends Connie or Sherrie or Carol will take care of you." And so on, forever.

Rx: Help them to help themselves. Persuade children to think of things they can do to make their stress more tolerable. Help them realize that disasters and traumas can be part of life, and that neither you, nor they, can always make bad things "go away." (And make sure you understand that you're not a "bad parent" because there is stress in their lives!) The sooner you can help them take responsibility for helping themselves cope with stress, the sooner they will feel more in control of those very situations that have made them feel out of control—and the sooner they will thank you.

Rx: Reassure your child about the safety precautions you're taking. If children are nervous, let them know you're doing everything in your power to keep them safe. Older children may be reassured by your honesty if you say you can't guarantee their safety but are doing everything you can think of to do.

Rx: Point out helpers and other "good" people—firefighters, police, doctors, nurses, rescue workers, and heroes. Be sure to observe out loud how many there are and how they outnumber any "bad guys." Encourage children to donate to relief groups, organize fund raisers, or volunteer to help in non traumatic rescue or cleanup efforts. Children can do more than just see the good guys—they can *be* the good guys. And you can support any dreams they may have of someday becoming a firefighter, police officer, doctor, nurse, rescue worker, or hero. Children love fantasy superheroes; it's a great gift to empower them with real-world dreams that might actually come true.

Rx: Encourage children to go back to school. Children generally feel fear for at least two weeks after a disaster or loss. They may become more clingy or whiny and are very likely to be afraid to leave you and go to school. It may seem to be very difficult advice for you, but guiding them back to school as soon as possible helps them gain needed perspective and overcome irrational fears. Returning to school is not just wise, it's crucial: If children avoid separating from you and feel a drop in their anxiety level when they cling, that drop will act like a reward for avoidance and will increase the chance that they will do it again and again. Gently encourage them to go back; go with them or find friends they can share their return with.

Rx: Use up the adrenaline. Make sure children have more than the usual opportunities to run, play, and move around. This will lead to less hypervigilance, hyperventilation, and hyperactivity later on.

Rx: Observe children objectively. If we see who children are rather than who we want them to be, we can quickly pick up how sensitive they are to stress. Then we can use that information to guide decisions about how to handle their stress.

Rx: Get outside help if necessary. Studies show that the sooner children get counseling after a catastrophic event, the less likely they will be to succumb later to Post-Traumatic Stress Disorder symptoms. (They're the same for children as for adults: nightmares, flashbacks, avoiding reminders of the disaster, apathy, trouble sleeping, irritability, poor concentration, jumpiness, and lack of faith in a bright future.) A survey of 12,000 children who survived a Hawaii hurricane found that those who got counseling early on were in better shape years later than those who didn't. Emotional stability, physical safety, and reliable grown-ups can't prevent disasters, but they can cultivate the resilience that protects children against its worst effects.

When a Parent Dies

For a child, the death of a parent is by far the most difficult disaster from which to recover, and it creates a wound that may never totally heal. The good news, however, is that few children show serious psychological disturbances in the years that follow, according to a Harvard University study of bereaved children. The loss of a parent affects a child in these understandable ways, all of which are normal reactions to an abnormal situation:

- They feel sad and miss the lost parent. Their grief will show up in psychological symptoms such as crying, trouble sleeping, and poor concentration.
- They'll express their emotional pain with minor physical ailments, such as colds, headaches, and stomachaches.
- They may feel guilty and wonder if they caused their parent's death by being "bad."
- They may feel angry about being abandoned, forced to move, or suddenly having less money if the parent who died was a major breadwinner.
- They may fret over the health of the remaining parent and go into a tailspin of worry over simple ailments such as colds or migraines.
- They may resent any "replacement spouse" and the new stepbrothers and stepsisters that come with him or her.

- They may stay connected to the lost parent through dreams, seeing the parent or hearing the parent's voice, feeling watched over by him or her, and imagining what heaven—where the parent is waiting—is like.
- They may weigh their behavior regarding whether it would have pleased the parent they lost.
- They may cling to belongings of the parent they lost as a way of staying connected.

By one year after the loss, however, time has usually begun to heal the wound—somewhat. In the Harvard study, psychologist William Worden and social work researcher Phyllis Silverman found most children cry less, sleep better, and can concentrate again, but headaches, stomachaches, and other physical problems still bother them as much as they did around the time of the loss.

Ways to help children get through the loss of a parent:

- Let them contribute to funeral arrangements or other mourning customs. Rituals dealing with death let people of all ages know that a community shares their grief. They also bring some small amount of *closure* (an ending, a significant passage).
- Let children talk about the dead parent. For now, they

need to keep the parent alive as they absorb their loss. Children may be better at talking about their lost loved one (who was real and touchable) than about their feelings (which are abstract). If it was the mother who died, children may have an especially deep need to connect and communicate. Losing a mother is often more difficult than losing a father, because of the amount of change that comes after a mother dies: The first touch you ever felt is gone, mealtimes may become less predictable, a different voice is reading the bedtime story, and someone less familiar is taking care of you when you get sick.

■ Let children maintain their daily routine as much as possible. The continuity of returning to the scene of the disaster and continuing with life as it was is reassuring and helps them rebuild the world into a safe place again.

■ Get help. A grieving spouse who tries to handle both his own grief and that of his children without any help is subjecting himself to cruel and unusual punishment! It's time to call in some support: Your children's grandparents, godparents, aunts, and uncles can all add nurturance to your own offerings to your children. Be sure, too, to allow children to turn to their friends, their friends' parents, and teachers for comfort. Many areas offer group grief counseling, also known as "bereavement" counseling. In these groups, children learn that others just like them share their experience and that they are not alone in their feelings.

Remember, even though disasters echo and symptoms persist, the history of the world shows us that with the right kind of models and support, children have the capacity to move forward and move beyond most trauma and loss. We can help most by showing them with our own lives that disaster is surmountable.

Chapter Twelve

Helping Others,
Helping Ourselves

We all know someone who needs StressRelief at this very minute—either because of a great disaster shared by the nation or a private disaster great or small. We all know someone who needs our help specifically or someone we particularly feel we need to help. The sad news is that so many are suffering from stress right now. The good news is that there is so much we can do to help.

SUPPORT RELIEF WORKERS

How can relief workers go into the debris of firestorms, the rubble of earthquakes, the ashes of airplane crashes, or Ground Zero after a terrorist attack and escape serious psychological symptoms? They can't. Relief workers often suffer from emotional numbness, flashbacks, sleep disturbances, depression, and concentration problems. In fact, many experts say at least one in every ten relief workers is suffering from Post-Traumatic Stress Disorder (PTSD) at any given time.

The most effective therapy for relief workers is group therapy. Police, firefighters, clergy, military, crisis counselors, medics, and EMS workers—they all need a turn to talk. But not to just anyone. They need an opportunity to talk to others who have been through the same nightmare, the same horrors, the same war. They need an opportunity to have others listen to whatever they have to say, no matter how gruesome, and not say anything in return—to just understand. No one can do that better than other relief workers!

This is a lesson for all of us. If you have been through a disaster, personal or public, reach out to others who shared the same experience—for your sake as well as for theirs. And follow these crisis intervention principles developed by specialists for helping relief workers manage their own stress:

1. **Call or visit** and let them know they're not alone!
2. **Let them talk!** Don't block, pacify, stop, or reject what they say. They are more likely to become depressed if they don't talk.
3. **Repeat what they've said.** This lets them know you were really listening, and gives them an opportunity to "hear" themselves and "listen to" themselves as they would another.
4. **Ask how they've tried to make themselves feel better or calmer.** Taking over or giving suggestions too soon may increase a sense of helplessness or frustration. Start with

their own plan of action (though many problems can't really be "solved") and ask how you can help.

5. **Set up a lot of follow-up.** Find other times to meet. Reassure them that they can call anytime. Discourage withdrawal from family or friends. Groups provide many more ears for listening and shoulders for support than a single counselor can ever offer.

6. **And stay in touch after relief efforts end!** That's when you'll be needed the most!

MOURNERS: WHAT TO SAY, WHAT NOT TO SAY

Soon after September 11, my neighbor told me that a co-worker lost his brother-in-law in the attack on the World Trade Center and that she had to pay a condolence call. "I don't know what to say," she said, "so I'm avoiding it."

"Actually," I reassured her, "you don't really have to say more than 'I'm sorry.' Just showing up or calling is enough." Survivors need company and an opportunity to talk, so listen. Here are the ABC's of sympathy:

- Acknowledge that something bad happened.
- Beware of clichés: They don't sound sincere.
- Console by saying, "I'm sorry." Researchers find that we want to hear those two words!

Then, if you want to say more, be specific and personal when you talk about the deceased. Describe one positive trait rather than making a list, and you'll sound like you mean it. Then let the mourner do the rest. And let the mourner know that the deceased not only loved them, but also felt loved *by* them! This will reduce the mourner's guilt and regrets.

Now, if you're in a similar situation and still feel you can't face the sorrow, or that a condolence call may stir up too much of your own sadness, write a note. The recipient can read and reread it at leisure and respond to it after having time to think. And stay in touch after the mourning period ends. That's when the true loneliness will set in.

THE GOOD FROM THE BAD

Trauma can change our behavior and beliefs. Great trauma can change our behavior and beliefs greatly. Since the terrorist attacks on September 11, polls find that 80 percent of us say we show more affection, 65 percent of us now see religion as very important (before the attack, 58 percent), and 65 percent of companies polled say employees are more caring toward one another. What I hear from callers to the FoxNews Channel when I have an open phone on air—and from my patients, friends, family, and colleagues at The Stress Program at Mount Sinai Hospital in New York—is that most of us are also rethinking how we spend our time. A few years ago, The Stress Program found that most of us are stressed by a *time deficit*—we're about twenty-one minutes short of the time we think we need every day. Until September 11, our family got leftover time. Now more of us are working at home to be near our family, scaling back hours, arranging for family mealtimes, attending our children's sports events, and even turning down promotions that would mean more time away from home.

And then there's our patriotism. How often have you heard that the attacks have given us patriotism once again? The truth, as I see it, is that we never lost our patriotism. We were never without it. The attacks have just brought it out more fully, helping us see it clearly and feel it dearly.

Disasters are not blessings in disguise. They are usually painful and frightening. Can we, however, find morals, lessons, and even slivers of silver linings? Of course. Do we have the capacity to survive and thrive? Yes. Do we have the capacity to grow and know when to take control, and when control is beyond us? Absolutely. Share the StressRelief Prescriptions and the list of mental health organizations provided by the National Institute of Mental Health that follow with those who need them—because we have the capacity to help ourselves and each other to StressRelief, and we do it best together!

167

The StressRelief
Prescriptions Checklist

If you have reached the end of this book and wish it went beyond one year—it does! As we know from the Myth of the Neat Stages, the StressRelief Prescriptions that appear at the end of each chapter can actually be used at any time—and they do their best work when you need them most. If your recovery is slow, if your pain level is high, or if you perhaps weren't ready for some of the prescriptions earlier, maybe they can help you now.

Most of the StressRelief Prescriptions have something in common: They employ Emotional CPR (Cognitive/Psychological Resuscitation). Remember that what we *think* and what we *do* will help shape what we *feel*, and this gives us power over our thoughts and behaviors. We can choose thoughts and behaviors that reinforce our sense of control. The good news is that you don't need someone else to apply Emotional CPR! All of the StressRelief Prescriptions that follow provide a means of giving Emotional CPR to yourself.

Here again are my StressRelief Prescriptions, plus other

advice from here and there in the preceding chapters—this time all in one place. Scan them to see if you missed any the first time through.

RELAX

Rx: Practice StressRelief Breathing. If your thinking is unclear, if shock is interfering with your ability to decide what to do next, or if you feel dizziness or other mild physical discomforts, force yourself to breathe slowly, in rhythm, from the belly, not the chest, pausing after each breath. This is the way babies breathe when they are sleeping. The reason you need lessons in this diaphragmatic breathing now is that, under disaster circumstances, we automatically breathe rapidly, which pushes carbon dioxide (CO_2) out of our lungs more quickly than normal. This hyperventilation may seem good at first, since CO_2 is the waste product of respiration, but this molecule does double duty. It's the collection of carbon dioxide in the bloodstream that is the signal to the brain that it's time to take the next breath. Not enough CO_2 because you've expelled so much? No need to take a breath, responds the brain. Soon you feel shortness of breath, dizziness, weakness, and tingling fingertips and lips, and you sweat. For some people, these symptoms are so uncomfortable that they create a panic attack, and that in turn makes the symptoms worse. You can stop the panic attack in twenty seconds to a minute by breathing slowly and pausing after every breath until the CO_2 builds up again and clear thinking returns.

If shallow panting is something you know you tend to do under stress, or if you do not know you tend to do it but experience the symptoms often, try this quick fix: Keep a small plastic or paper bag with you and breathe into and out of it when you feel short of breath. This will rapidly increase your CO_2 level. Then you can begin StressRelief Breathing to clear your head. Practice now—and in the car, in line at the market, and during a long elevator ride. Count back from ten to one, and take a gentle breath on each count. Let the air fill your belly when you breathe in. Then gently exhale, relax, and pause a beat. Try to relax more and more on each count. When you've become practiced, do a second set with your eyes closed if practical. Or pretend that your breath is a mist of your favorite color so that you create more and more of a mist of this color when you exhale. The imagery will involve your right hemisphere and give you some relief from the worrying centered in your left hemisphere.

Rx: Take breaks. A total of twenty minutes of StressRelief a day is enough to decrease stress symptoms and improve your mood, according to research by Herbert Benson, M.D., of Harvard University. That's a *total* of twenty minutes. Two minutes of breathing exercises in a stuck elevator, four minutes of Progressive Muscle Relaxation on a long line, or fifteen minutes of walking or meditation all count toward the total. The effect of these breaks is to help reduce adrenaline production . . . and prevent the insomnia, headaches, stomach upsets, and other distur-

170

bances that may linger for years unless we do something about them now. In fact, many studies have found that hormones produced under stress suppress the number of certain blood cells that protect us against infections and cancers. This may help to explain why widows and widowers are at higher risk of illness for the first two months after the death of a spouse, why stress precedes sore throats and colds four times more frequently than it follows them, and why women under the chronic stress of caring for parents with Alzheimer's disease show reduced immune functioning.

Bottom line: We can't fight chronic stress and still fight illness efficiently. So if you think you can't afford to schedule downtime right now, consider this: Without twenty minutes of downtime a day *by choice*, you're likely to have more downtime later *without choice* because of stress symptoms—lying in a darkened room with a migraine, lying awake at night with insomnia, or immobilized by stomachaches or back pains. Take breaks right now from rescue efforts, daily demands, or even mourning, and you'll increase your sense of control and decrease your recovery time.

Rx: Pause five times a day. One good way to reach and exceed the recommended twenty minutes of StressRelief each day is to take five breaks a day of five minutes each. This can cut stress symptoms in half, according to research. Use the breaks in any way that turns off your fight-or-flight response: phone a friend;

do a crossword puzzle; listen to music; browse a bookstore; get a backrub; say a prayer; clean your wallet; play with a child; repot a plant; pet a pet; take a walk; think of yourself as a camera and savor the image of someone being helpful, something unusual, or whatever pleases your mind's eye; or try a relaxation exercise such as StressRelief Breathing, autohypnosis, or Progressive Muscle Relaxation.

Rx: Try Progressive Muscle Relaxation. This simple exercise is great for counteracting tension. Some of my patients make a tape of their own voice giving the following instructions:

1. Starting with the toes, and relax.
2. Then the feet and ankles: relax.
3. Then the calves: relax.
4. The knees: relax.
5. The thighs: relax.
6. The buttocks: relax.
7. The abdomen and stomach: relax.
8. The back and shoulders: relax.
9. The hands: relax.
10. The forearms: relax.
11. The upper arms: relax.
12. The neck: relax.
13. The face: relax.
14. Now, drift off.

You can also begin to counteract tension with the following technique: Slowly contract and relax each part of your body for ten seconds each. Then, contract and relax each part of your body more quickly to become aware of the tension/relaxation contrast.

Rx: Hypnotize yourself. Let your body know it's time to relax with this classic autohypnosis exercise from Stanley Fisher, Ph.D., author of *Discovering the Power of Self-Hypnosis: The Simple, Natural Mind-Body Approach to Change and Healing*:

1. Sit comfortably in a chair facing a wall about eight feet away. Pick a spot or an object on the wall about a foot above your sitting eye level. This is your focal point.
2. Look at your focal point and begin counting backward from 100, one number for each breath you exhale.
3. As you count and continue to concentrate on your focal point, imagine yourself floating, floating down—down through the chair—very relaxed.
4. As you stare at the focal point, you will find that your eyelids feel heavier and begin to blink. When this happens, just let your eyes slowly close.
5. While your eyes are closed, continue to count backward— one number for each time you exhale. As you count, imagine how it would feel to be as limp as a rag doll, totally relaxed and floating in a safe, comfortable space. This is your space.

6. As that safe, comfortable feeling flows over you, stop counting and just float.
7. If any disturbing thoughts enter your space, just let them flow out again; continue to feel safe and relaxed.
8. To come out of autohypnosis, either let yourself drift off to sleep, or count to three and exit using the following steps: At one, let yourself get ready; at two, take a deep breath and hold it for a few seconds; at three, exhale and open your eyes slowly. As you open your eyes, continue to hold on to that relaxed, comfortable feeling.

Rx: Play. What movies came out lately? Which sports teams are ahead, what music groups have had hits, and what shows are big on Broadway or on TV? What games did your child, niece, or nephew get for a recent birthday, and do the new swings at the playground need a test drive? If you don't know, it's time to find out. Young people provide special opportunities for fun. But putting the play back in your life can actually be more than fun—it's healthful. An Israeli study showed that young people who distracted themselves with games or caring for others during a disaster were less likely to suffer from Post-Traumatic Stress Disorder (PTSD) than those who closely monitored news reports about the disaster.

Rx: Bore yourself to sleep. If you can't sleep because your brain is on alert after an unexpected trauma, one way to find

174

StressRelief from hypervigilance is to flood the brain with the predictable. Follow your regular bedtime routine so you know exactly what's coming next. Turn on your favorite music so you know every note. Rock yourself like a baby so your body knows every motion. And then lull your brain to sleep with easy, repetitive prayers, poems, nursery rhymes, or even by counting sheep. The familiar words and repeated rhythms help to quiet the stress response.

Rx: Use meditation or prayer. If you awaken during the night, try reciting a prayer, poem, comforting phrase, or mantra. The familiar words and repeated rhythms help to quiet the stress response and reassure our brain that the world is predictable. Soothing thoughts soothe the emotions.

TAKE ACTION

Rx: Talk to yourself! If others remind you that things could be worse, their efforts are not likely to have an effect. But research finds that our mood does lift when we give *ourselves* the same pep talk. So do it! Focus on the positive and remind yourself that there is still much for which we can be thankful.

Rx: Do something physical. If you are hyperactive and overenergized, you'll need to get rid of some of that adrenaline before you can truly rest. Run around the house until you have used up some of the adrenaline and feel your energy level come down—or until you have to stop! Put on music with a beat faster than your heartbeat—about 72 beats per minute—and run in place. You'll able to relax once the adrenaline has burned off.

Rx: Get back to basics. Choose to get back to dealing with daily demands. Stock up, fix up, pick up, and repair. Filling the refrigerator, picking up children's clothes, or picking up a hammer restores our sense of control. We may not be able to solve the anthrax problem or prevent earthquakes, but we can clean a kitchen drawer and reorganize our wallet—and our brain reacts as if order has been brought to the world for now. Getting back to basics also brings us into contact with others, and the interactions are usually reassuring. We get to see others going about daily tasks, gather information or sympathy or support, feel less isolated, and are reminded of the roles we fill and why we are needed. Going back to basics does not mean that we are disrespecting a parent who died or a colleague we lost. It means we are programmed to move out of suspended animation and take care of business to insure our own survival—not just physical survival, but psychological survival as well.

Rx: Volunteer. If there's been a major disaster and you're still on your feet, you are needed. Volunteer to help. Volunteering will show you that although you've had losses, you still have something to give; although you feel drained, you still have strength.

And volunteering seems to help your health. Allan Luks, author of *The Healing Power of Doing Good*, finds that people who volunteer weekly are ten times more likely to say they're healthy than people who volunteer only once a year. The volunteers report fewer headaches and backaches and less arthritis pain, possibly because nurturing behavior may flood us with endorphins, the body's natural painkillers.

Rx: Take one task at a time. Before the disaster, you may have been a multitasker and even loved having many balls in the air at once. But now, you may be so distracted and processing so much new information that one ball is all you can handle. Your concentration isn't very good right now, and trying to do more than one task at a time may mean you start everything, finish nothing, and make errors as well. This will only increase your sense of frustration and your stress level. Choosing one job and making a small amount of solid progress, on the other hand, will restore your sense of control.

Rx: Stick with routines and schedules. Familiar patterns—regular mealtimes, weekly activities, the ever-reliable school bell—are reassuring, particularly to children and the vulnerable elderly. One might think that children wouldn't have a severe reaction since they seem to be less aware of events, but in my work for my book *KidStress*, I found the cue for child stress is grown-up stress—from teachers and parents on down to older siblings. As for the elderly, we assume that because they have lived longer they're more philosophical, but their pain may be even greater since they may have lived through many disasters before . . . and those memories may return full force now. Routines and schedules provide the security they need.

Rx: Add bedtime predictability. Bedtimes are especially important, because for every hour that our sleep pattern is thrown off, it usually takes twenty-four hours for the body to readjust. So even if you feel a disaster has wrecked your schedule completely and even if all you want to do is eat and sleep, push yourself to get up at the same time every morning—on the early side if possible. Remember, the body needs early morning light to reset its biological clock each day. When you wake up tired, plan to go to bed earlier tonight rather than sleeping in now.

Rx: Prioritize. We may feel bogged down by all the small things that aren't getting done, but there are some bigger issues to consider:

1. **Check your physical health.** Wear and tear often doesn't show up until months after an emergency—so late that we may not even suspect that ailments are disaster-related.
2. **Check your emotional health.** If the Three G's (guilt, grief, or grim predictions) or depression are the emotion of the day—every day—see a counselor or a physician for a referral.

3. **Check loved ones' physical health.** Are they ailing bodily? Are they refusing invitations for reasons of illness or physical discomfort? Do what you can to help and heal.
4. **Check loved ones' emotional health.** Have people you know dropped out of social interactions? Are they depressed? Again, see that they get help.

UNDERSTAND AND ACCEPT YOURSELF

Rx: Accept your emotions. Whatever your emotions are after a disaster, you have enough to worry about without having to worry that your reactions are something to worry about!

According to many researchers, 90 percent of us will begin to feel stressed or shocked by the end of Day One. Ninety percent is most but not all of us. Some may bypass shock altogether (most likely those trained for emergencies), and some will feel stress long before the end of Day One. All are normal reactions to an abnormal situation. Rather than fear that your numbness means you are unfeeling, observe it with interest and know that it is protecting you from thoughts you cannot accept just yet. Rather than being horrified by the reckless risk you took to help someone, try to be amazed at your impulse to heroism.

Rx: Know that StressRelief takes time. Soon after the first shock wave of the disaster response has crested and passed, there may be smaller second and third waves—or more disasters that start up our reactions all over again. Remember that the brain can process new information only so fast, and each of us will work through our thoughts and emotions at our own individual, personal pace. You may feel a tiny bit better today . . . and tomorrow you will add to that foundation of feeling and healing.

Rx: Remind yourself that anniversary reactions are normal and temporary—and may even be part of your healing. After the anniversary—which can come a week later, a month later, a year later, or many years in the future—you'll probably pick up where you left off, and you may even be stronger. If being in a certain place at a certain time triggers memories, arrange to be in a different place on the next anniversary. Removing yourself physically can separate you from many of the cues that will trigger an uncomfortable reaction.

PUT IT ON PAPER

Rx: Make a list. Committing our thoughts to paper can mean we no longer need to keep them in our heads, where they'll bother us. So:

1. Pull out a pencil and make a list of what has to be done to deal with the disaster.
2. Add everything that didn't get done because of the disaster.

3. Add items for tomorrow, next week, and next month if you can think that far ahead.

This simple list will help you focus on the near future, ground yourself with a plan, replace the sense of uselessness with a sense of purpose, and remind yourself that you have a "village brain"— that you are a needed member of a family and larger community. After all, one reason you are suffering now is that you care for others. They care for you, too!

Rx: Take an inventory. Disaster victims may say that they're still not over it, that they're still suffering, that they're still mourning, or that not a day goes by that they don't think about it. But when a therapist, counselor, or family member looks at certain specifics (see the list below), it turns out that the victim has made progress without realizing it. If you feel stalled—or if an Anniversary Reaction has set you back—place a check mark by the statements that are true for you now and see how far you've come:

___ StressRelief exercises have calmed me since the disaster.
___ Prayer or meditation have helped me feel better since the disaster.
___ I've taken part in ceremonies, observances, or other group activities since the disaster.
___ Substance problems or addictions had a grip on me— until I got a grip on them.

___ Fears and phobias were running my life—until I got help and demystified them.

___ Physical problems threatened to overwhelm me—until I saw a doctor, made a plan, or took action.

___ I've stopped blaming myself for what happened.

___ I sleep much better than I did right after the disaster.

___ My dreams and flashbacks don't seem strange to me now.

___ I talk about my dreams and flashbacks with others.

___ Grief and pain are still with me, but they're not as acute or constant as they were before.

___ I've accepted invitations to go places and do things since the disaster.

___ I've extended invitations to friends and acquaintances since the disaster.

___ I smile much more than I did at first.

___ I've caught myself laughing since the disaster.

___ I have actually had some fun since the disaster.

Scoring: If you marked *any* of the statements in the checklist above, you've taken a big step toward recovery. Read the unchecked statements again for ideas about what steps to take next.

REACH OUT

Rx: Talk. As the shock begins to wear off, those of us who have had a direct loss—a parent, child, friend, or colleague—will be going through acute stress and grief. We will be hit over and over by waves of pain, and we may hear ourselves sighing. The world will seem unreal—and one of the best ways to reconnect is to talk, talk, talk. If there's no one to talk to, look for someone—ask for a counselor or go to religious services or family gatherings. Why do experts advise talking after every crisis—national or personal? Because talking gives us:

- A sense of *doing* something
- An opportunity to *hear* ourselves
- A chance to *listen* to ourselves as others would
- An opportunity to adjust our thoughts and feelings
- A chance to better understand what we're thinking or feeling

Besides, most feelings are less ominous when they are said out loud to others in the light of day than when they are silently thought, alone, in the middle of the night.

Rx: Take part in ceremony and ritual. Holding candles and singing with others in a vigil, attending a "town meeting" where people can talk and cry together, or presenting donations collected in a huge fund-raiser can bring us closer, and all are a great antidote to depression because they remind us that coming together in times of trauma is something we do naturally. Even mourning rituals, like funerals, can give us needed closure and remind us that we are supported and cared for. Try joining or organizing such a group or activity, such as those around the country that followed September 11:

- Church and school bells ringing in unison
- Candles flickering at every street corner
- Patriotic hymns in karaoke bars
- Special services in houses of worship
- Moments of silence
- Concerts and sing-ins
- College and university chapel services and symposia on issues raised by the disaster
- Prayer vigils
- Poetry readings and music
- Parades of police cars and fire trucks
- A day of reflection in schools, featuring readings, art creations, and performances

Rx: Connect. You may be tempted to unplug the phone, pull down the shades, and slide deep under the covers, but don't. Perhaps you can't do anything to change the personal or national disaster you just suffered, but you *can* help family and friends, and they can help you. Because we all have a "village brain," we do better when we see others face to face. Just as the youngest baby is programmed to smile at us and make us smile back—and form a bond—we're all programmed to take care of each other. Even if you don't know what to do to make yourself feel better, others may have ideas for getting your daily life back to normal. If you're mildly shocked or having symptoms of Emotionally-Toxic Shock, people around you can pick up signs you can't pick up in yourself. Provide yourself with opportunities to behave normally, to reengage, and to increase your sense of control. Reach out to the people who are important in your life, share your experiences, and feel yourself reactivate in response to others. Lunch appointments, dinner plans, holiday family gatherings, movies, and sports (both those played and those watched) are all opportunities to consider instead of turn down. Later, the re-emerging interest in sex is another step in recovery, since satisfying sex increases endorphins, which are natural mood elevators and painkillers; scrotonin, a calm-down, feel-good brain chemical; dopamine, which suppresses appetite; and several more.

Rx: Don't substitute the media for real people. Though the radio seems like a companion and the television seems like a friendly presence, their messages and images have the power to cause pain, and they will never respond to you. Real people—face to face will. They will help you feel more connected, listen to your thoughts and fears, and share your concerns.

Rx: Don't be afraid to talk about dreams and flashbacks. The repetition in dreams and flashbacks helps desensitize us to the disaster. The thoughts and feelings of dreams and flashbacks will be less frightening in the light of day than in the middle of the night when we're alone and waking up in a cold sweat. Furthermore, when we allow ourselves to talk about dreams and flashbacks, we give others around us permission to talk about theirs. We're reassuring them that their experience is not uncommon and giving them an opportunity to reassure us of the same thing.

Rx: Celebrate. Weddings, charity functions, and patriotic events are all legitimate and may be attended with relief and pleasure because it is still possible to do something so normal. For those who feel ready and able, holidays can be celebrated with gusto—even by those of us who are still grieving. And we're often ready to think about taking a vacation again.

Rx: Handle the holidays. There are a number of ways to make sure holidays are the joyful events they should be:

- **Plan time with family or friends who are nurturing, welcoming, and happy.** Spend as little face time as possible with those who are not.
- **Create one or two new traditions to mark this holiday as different.** That way you'll be less apt to compare it to the past.
- **Keep it low key.** A quiet, meaningful celebration is what many disaster survivors want and need.

- **Be realistic.** Don't expect a picture-perfect holiday celebration this year. It was never picture-perfect in the past—why should it be now? Lines for gift-wrapping won't be faster, airport security screening won't disappear, and Uncle Henry is not going to be friendlier this year. Focus on what you can control, like good food, music, and company.
- **Converse with constraints.** Discuss, don't debate; communicate to be heard, not to win; share information and facts, not opinions and angry words and focus on the future with hope and try not to look back with nostalgia.
- **Don't compare your holidays to anyone else's,** and stop thinking that yours are not good enough. That is mental cruelty and probably inaccurate anyway.
- **Avoid overeating, overdrinking, oversmoking, and overspending.** Getting a grip will give a needed sense of control.
- **Pause often.** Time may be tight, but we all need a break from adrenaline. Massages and yoga classes make great gifts—for others and also for yourself.
- **Attend religious or spiritual services.** The familiarity, rhythmic chanting, gathering of congregations, and meditation time are all stress relievers.
- **Remember that celebrating holidays is natural.** Holidays are life-focused, good for children, and a way of bonding with family and community.

CHANGE YOUR MIND

Rx: Behave "as if." Even if the "To Do" list seems irrelevant now, we can behave "as if" it's important to us and *do it anyway!* This is a basic principle of Emotional CPR. By behaving "as if" life is normalized, we're putting ourselves into situations that will help move us in that direction and increase the odds of soon feeling "as if," as well. We begin to interact with people we wouldn't have been with otherwise, get feedback we wouldn't have gotten otherwise, and feel new demands on ourselves which can make us feel needed, vital, and alive. If we behave as if our feelings are more normalized, pretty soon they will be:

- When you feel anxious, behave "as if" you feel more calm. Soon your brain will follow your behavior into a calmer state of mind.
- When you're feeling apathetic, act "as if" you want to get up and take care of the yard work or project. Since you have probably had a better attitude about the yard work or project in the past, the old feeling may come back in the environment where the accomplishment is to take place.
- When you're feeling asocial, like crawling into a cave by yourself and hibernating for years, force yourself to get out and do some socializing. It will distract you and probably spark a new series of invitations and friendships. They will, in turn, pull you out of the cave and into the sunlight.

188

*Rx: **Plan for the Six D's.*** If distraction, disorganization, depression, destabilization, decision-making difficulties, and dependency fantasies crop up now, take a breath, pause, and try again. And don't blame yourself. Putting yourself down won't get the e-mail done or help you figure out where you parked the car.

*Rx: **Demystify fears and phobias.*** If you're overwhelmed by phobias and irrational fears, talk to yourself using the words you imagine a logical, levelheaded friend would use: "You know it's extremely unlikely that another hurricane this destructive will come during your lifetime" and "You know it's extremely unlikely that you'll be mugged again." If a gray sky or dark street give you a sense of foreboding, observe that most of the time, gentle showers come from gray skies and people are probably sleeping peacefully inside the homes lining dark streets. If the sound of an airplane makes you hunch your shoulders defensively, observe that the vast majority of the time, airplanes are carrying not terrorists but vacationers and businesspeople to their destinations. This kind of talk therapy can actually begin to reverse the biochemical processes that cause fears and phobias (though in severe cases, pharmacological help may be needed).

*Rx: **Forgive yourself.*** Instead of creating escape fantasies in which you stop the disaster and save lives, berating yourself for your last irritable words to someone who never came home, or feeling guilty, forgive yourself the way you know other people would forgive you if they could. We can only do what we can do at a given moment; we only know what we know; and if we made a mistake, that's what we have to live with. Self-blame stands in the way of acceptance and normal life—by forgiving ourselves, we accept our true limitations.

Rx: Give yourself permission to feel better. It's possible that you may have mixed feelings about allowing yourself to heal. When the pain lets up, it raises distressing questions about how deeply you really cared about the losses of the disaster. Don't worry! When pain starts to let up, it doesn't mean you're insensitive; it means you allowed yourself to feel your feelings fully, have moved through them, and are beginning to come out on the other side.

Rx: Don't confuse the acute pain and initial anxiety with sadness. If you think you will always feel this bad, you have not been through a disaster before. Pain and anxiety do let up eventually. Sadness, on the other hand, is a feeling that can, and often does, last forever. This doesn't mean we can't experience joy, love, and excitement. But unlike the acute pain and initial anxiety, which fade, the sadness when we do think about the disaster may always be there.

Rx: Don't be afraid to laugh. The first jokes we hear after a major disaster may strike us as tasteless or disrespectful, but they do have a purpose: Laughter is a natural StressRelief mechanism. We are not callous; we are alive. The smaller the disaster, the sooner the jokes will start. And if the disaster was, for example, all the computers going down at the bank, the jokes could start that day since losses were digital, not human. So enjoy the laughter. It releases the body's own stress-reducing biochemicals, and it blocks anxiety and fear.

Rx: *Distract yourself.* You don't have to watch all the TV coverage of a disaster, keep the radio on 24/7, or attend every memorial service. Choose one or two meaningful observances and then find something else to do. Movies work well, many say, because they replace the thoughts and sounds in our heads with fresh dialogue, music, and new images.

Rx: Try cinema therapy. After the September 11 attacks, restaurant revenue went down, but Americans apparently spent more money at the movies than at any time since World War II. Moviegoers paid nearly $100 million to see *Harry Potter and the Sorcerer's Stone* in its first weekend two months after the tragedy. It's possible that the film would have been a huge hit without the tragedies, but it didn't hurt that it had for its theme a mysterious, alien, evil force conquered by children who are kind, brave, persistent, and pure of heart. Because of this universal theme, it's also possible that parents nobly taking their children to see Harry Potter got something out of the movie, too.

Movies are more than just entertainment. In times of transition or uncertainty, scary images from our real life are replaced by movie images we know are make-believe. We can lose ourselves for a few hours, and there are no announcers cutting in with bad news. If the movie is the first in a series, it promises a future we can look forward to. At the movie house, we come together for a safe emotional experience with other people, hear the laughter, and share the tears. Movies can make us feel better—cinema therapy—and during tough times, here are the categories that relieve stress best:

- **Comfort movies.** These films are so familiar we can recite almost every line; because of this predictability, the brain goes off alert and relaxes. Some examples: *Grease* (if you were alive in the seventies, you know every song!), *The Godfather* (the guys in my family know every word!).

- **Classic war movies.** These remind us that we've been through difficult times before and came out on top. Try *Casablanca* (tough guy becomes patriotic and noble) or *Mutiny on the Bounty*.

- **Family movies.** The movies in this group make us feel cozy and reminiscent. Classics are *The Sound of Music* (a true story about a family that escapes World War II and, by the way, ended up in the United States) and *It's a Wonderful Life* (perhaps one of the most uplifting movies of all time, one that reminds us of the value of community).

- **Movies with humor.** Laughter is nature's antidote to stress—so use it! Recent favorites, according to box office reports, are *There's Something About Mary* (painfully funny, as one reviewer put it) and *Home Alone* (kids find this one real StressRelief).

Rx: Be open to the new view. At some point after a disaster, we may look back on the event and suddenly find that it somehow looks different, a phenomenon called "reframing." What once seemed to us to be a very personal event may suddenly take on political significance now. We may find that we have learned beneficial lessons from the trauma or may have a more realistic view about how uncommon this kind of disaster is.

Rx: Review lessons learned. The aftermath of the attacks of September 11, 2001, was a lesson in kindness, generosity, and forward motion that we can take with us into the future:

- Rescue workers traveled thousands of miles to volunteer their help free of charge. They then willingly stood in line for hours waiting for their assignments.
- So much donated food and clothing poured into New York that rescue workers couldn't use it all, and some of it had to be warehoused.
- Millions of Americans donated so much blood that the Red Cross had more than it could use at the time.
- Americans gave $1.2 billion to charities formed to help disaster victims and their families.

- Strangers held hands and sang together at candlelight vigils across the country.
- Relationships were rekindled as we looked up old friends to ask if they were okay.
- And business at one New York-area dating service doubled as singles began to realize how much can happen in a day.

Rx: Don't confuse the anniversary reaction with depression or seasonal blahs. It's easy to assume that feeling down or "off" relates to spring hay fever, fall allergies, the start of school, waning winter light (a winter blues condition called Seasonal Affective Disorder), or just plain depression. But if negative feelings seem to come and go on a regular basis, make a note of the month, day, or condition of their onset because you may be having an Anniversary Reaction. Does it relate in some way to the month, day, or condition of a disaster in the past? If so, you now know why the antihistamines or light therapy didn't work. You can begin now to treat the symptoms with the right "medicine"— and get real StressRelief.

Rx: Listen, listen, listen. If someone has had a direct loss, be ready to listen, listen, listen! Repeat back what they say so they know you heard every word and that none of them are too dreadful to be said out loud. It's wise to avoid clichés such as "I know how you feel . . . " unless you have had a similar loss and really do know! A simple "I'm sorry" tends to be what brings the most comfort to the most people. It's important to reassure all talkers that you'll be there long after the press has left and relief services have gone. Children and the elderly especially tend to be lost in the shuffle.

Rx: Hang around optimists. If the future seems empty and apathy is the mood, choose your companions wisely! Make a conscious effort to surround yourself with optimism and relaxation, and avoid a lot of face-to-face time with people who are "down." This doesn't mean you should suddenly shed all stressed friends. But attitudes are contagious; if you find yourself at an emotional low point, try to balance the stressed friends with an equal-sized group of people who are action-oriented.

GET HELP

Rx: Get professional help. If daily life has lost its rhythm, if your personality seems changed rather than just shaken up, if physical or psychological symptoms are not abating, and if you're feeling alone and unable to help yourself, this is not the time to tough it out. You probably have plenty of resources: friends, family, clergy, and professional counselors. By talking to others and by sharing and comparing your experiences and reactions, you may find that your thoughts are not too extreme to express after all.

Rx: Consider group therapy. Another option is to find a *group* of others who feel the same way you do. The one in ten relief workers who suffer from Post-Traumatic Stress Disorder (PTSD) after a disaster are generally offered group crisis intervention. Family physicians and religious leaders are good sources for support groups. Research finds groups even more effective than individual therapists for this kind of post-traumatic reaction. Trauma victims need people to listen, respond, and sympathize—and the more listeners in the group, the more response and sympathy are available. In a group, ideas tend to flow and concepts of all kinds are voiced—and found to be common, benign, and more manageable than they seemed in the middle of the night. In fact, someone in the group may be a perfect match for our own experience and feelings. Consider that just about any group, even one not led by a professional counselor, can be full of "therapists" who can help you—wise friends, sympathetic family members, colleagues, and fellow congregants. The time and expense of group therapy is usually less than that of individual therapy, but if symptoms don't go away, the hours and cost of individual therapy may be well worth it.

Rx: Get professional help if the holidays are more burden than blessing. Watch for these trouble signs:

- Loss of appetite
- Increased isolation
- Difficulty falling asleep or staying asleep
- Agitated or slowed-down behavior

- Constant fatigue
- Sadness
- Difficulty thinking or concentrating

Rx: Get help from family. A grieving spouse who tries to handle both his own grief and that of his children without some help is subjecting himself to cruel and unusual punishment! It's time to call in some support: Your children's grandparents, godparents, aunts, and uncles can all add nurturance to your own offerings to your children. Be sure, too, to allow children to turn to their friends, their friends' parents, and teachers for comfort. Many areas offer group "bereavement" counseling. In these groups, children learn that others just like them share their experience and that they are not alone in their grief.

Rx: Get outside help for children if necessary. Studies show that the sooner children get counseling after a catastrophic event, the less likely they will be to succumb later to PTSD symptoms. (The symptoms are the same for children as for adults: nightmares, flashbacks, avoiding reminders of the disaster, apathy, trouble sleeping, irritability, poor concentration, jumpiness, and lack of faith in a bright future.) A survey of 12,000 children who survived a Hawaii hurricane found that those who got counseling early on were in better shape years later than those who didn't. Emotional stability, physical safety, and reliable grown-ups can't prevent disasters, but they can cultivate the resilience that protects children against its worst effects.

Rx: For anniversary reactions, find a support group, or see your therapist more often. The support group for survivors of a major Virginia flood in November 1985 sponsored a covered-dish supper in a church a few days before the anniversary of the flood. On the anniversary evening, the group also encouraged residents to put lighted candles in their front windows, which served, in the words of one survivor, as "a memorial to those who died in the flood, as a tribute to those who worked in flood relief, and as a symbol for the undying spirit of those who have survived the flood." The large community response was heartwarming and healing. If the anniversary reaction hits so hard it flattens you, you may need outside help. Though the reaction usually fades within days, those days can be unbearable for some. If the reaction goes on and on, a therapist can help you sort out the cause.

HELP OTHERS

Rx: Reach out to those who are grieving. If a friend has had a loss, try helping in the following ways:

- **Allow her to formulate her own alternatives** without overwhelming her with advice or threatening her sense of self-confidence.
- **Do not deny his sorrow and loss.** Reminding him that the person he's grieving for had a good life or died without pain won't help his separation anxiety and may make him feel guilty for thinking of himself.

- **Don't stay away.** Although she may be withdrawn, upset, or proud, even silent company offers security.
- **Offer social and work activities without pressure.** Don't try to guess what is appropriate for him; everyone handles reengagement differently. Let him know that he's welcome to join life rather than being left to mimic death. It doesn't imply disrespect for his loss when he functions as fully as he can.

Rx: Let children contribute to funeral arrangements or other mourning customs. Rituals dealing with death let people of all ages know that a community shares their grief. They also bring some small amount of *closure* (an ending, a significant passage).

Rx: Let children talk about the dead parent. For now, they need to keep the parent alive as they absorb their loss. Children may be better at talking about their lost loved one (who was real and touchable) than about their feelings (which are abstract). If it was the mother who died, children may have an especially deep need to connect and communicate. Losing a mother is often more difficult than losing a father, because of the amount of change that comes after a mother dies: The first touch you ever felt is gone, mealtimes may become less predictable, a different voice is reading the bedtime story, and someone less familiar is taking care of you when you are sick.

Rx: Child-size the disaster. Explain the disaster to children in the simplest, most reassuring terms you can. Let them know how they are being protected. Find some activities to "make things better": Draw pictures as gifts for the bereaved, make food for those in shelters, and so forth. You don't have to explain every detail about the disaster to your child. It may be more than they want to know or need to know, and it may make the stress much worse. And it's not a good idea for them to see disaster images again and again on television. If they are very young, they will think that it has happened many times.

Rx: Don't shield children totally. You may be tempted to call a moratorium on the news or unplug the TV, but if the children in your life are school-age, they'll find out anyway.

Rx: Ask children lots of questions. Have a family discussion in which everyone (including you) is encouraged to say how he or she feels. To get the conversation started, you can ask, "What do you think happened?" or "If you were the President, what would you do?" Listen to all answers and repeat them back to show you heard every word. Children may then qualify or change their statements, which means you've provoked thoughtfulness. When they ask the same question over and over, smile . . . and know that this is their way of digesting tough information. Be on the look-out for physical signs of stress in your children, who don't have the words to express their new feelings of fear: stomachaches, headaches, too much eating or not enough, nightmares, and dis-tractibility.

Rx: Understand that children don't understand. Children can comprehend only experiences they have had themselves. A six-year-old who has never had a relative pass away may think that disaster victims are only sleeping. Even teens may not think logically, fantasizing, for example, that a deceased parent will somehow come back.

Rx: Remind children of the "chain of love." A disaster can stir up fears of losing a parent for the first time, and the experience can leave a child feeling small and alone. One of the best antidotes (for adults, too) is what I call the "the chain of love": "If anything happens to Mommy, Daddy is right here to take care of you. If anything happens to Daddy, Grandma and Grandpa love you and will take care of you. If anything happens to Grandma and Grandpa, Aunt Gretchen loves you and will take care of you. If anything happens to Aunt Gretchen, Mommy's best friends Connie or Sherrie or Carol will take care of you." And so on, forever.

Rx: Help children help themselves. Persuade children to think of things they can do to make their stress more tolerable. Help them realize that disasters and traumas can be part of life, and that neither you, nor they, can always make bad things "go away." (And make sure you understand that you're not a "bad parent" because there is stress in their lives!) The sooner you can help them take responsibility for helping themselves cope with stress, the sooner they will feel more in control of those very situations that have made them feel out of control. And the sooner they will thank you.

Rx: Reassure children about the safety precautions you're taking. If children are nervous, let them know you're doing everything in your power to keep them safe. Older children may be reassured by your honesty if you say you can't guarantee their safety but are doing everything you can think of to do.

Rx: Point out helpers and other "good" people—firefighters, police, doctors, nurses, rescue workers, and heroes. Be sure to observe out loud how many there are and how they outnumber any "bad guys." Encourage children to donate to relief groups, organize fundraisers, or volunteer to help in nontraumatic rescue or cleanup efforts. Children can do more than just see the good guys—they can *be* the good guys. And you can support any dreams they may have of someday becoming a firefighter, police officer, doctor, nurse, rescue worker, or hero. Children love fantasy superheroes; it's a great gift to empower them with real-world dreams that might actually come true.

Rx: Encourage children to go back to school. Children generally feel fear for at least two weeks after a disaster or loss. They may become more clingy or whiny and are very likely to be afraid to leave you and go to school. It may seem to be very difficult advice for you, but guiding them back to school as soon as possible helps them gain needed perspective and overcome irrational fears. Returning to school is not just wise, it's crucial: If children avoid separating from you and feel a drop in their anxiety level when they cling, that drop will act like a reward for avoidance and will increase the chance that they will do it again and again. Gently encourage them to go back; go with them or find friends they can share their return with.

Rx: Use up the adrenaline. Make sure children have more than the usual opportunities to run, play, and move around. This will lead to less hypervigilance, hyperventilation, and hyperactivity later on.

Rx: Observe children objectively. If we see who children are rather than who we want them to be, we can quickly pick up how sensitive they are to stress. Then we can use that information to guide decisions about how to handle their stress.

MONITOR YOUR BODY

Rx: See your doctor for medical concerns. If chronic digestive problems develop, if existing problems such as irritable bowel syndrome (IBS), migraine headaches, or allergies suddenly get much worse, if the menstrual cycle becomes erratic, or if any unexplained symptoms appear, see a doctor. He or she may not only be able to help prevent chronic problems but can make suggestions about psychological or spiritual counseling if needed.

Rx: Maintain healthy habits. Though many Americans began to throw caution to the winds and feasted on wine, cheesecake, and other caloric delicacies after the terrorist attacks of September 11, Bruce McEwen, Ph.D., of The Rockefeller University in New York, reminds us that such indulgence is dangerous under stressful conditions: Prolonged stress usually changes patterns of living, including eating more high-fat food, sleeping badly, skipping exercise, or drinking more, he says. These in turn cause changes in the stress hormones, which in turn increase our risk of heart disease, depression, and some types of cancer. The setting may have changed, but the risks have not! By neglecting or abusing ourselves now, we are setting ourselves up for more stress in the future. This is a time to give ourselves as much care as always—maybe even more.

Rx: Announce your intention to kick addictions. A disaster can often lead us into unwanted addictions, or worsen an addiction we already had. Once you make the decision, broadcast the news that you're about to dump your addictions and break your bad habits. Tell the world you're going to quit smoking, stop using drugs, and not eat or drink so much anymore. If you can't keep yourself honest, let the world help. No excuses! Get tough now, since problems tend to grow, not dwindle. A specialist can guide you though cognitive therapy, behavioral therapy, group therapy, or medication if necessary.

Rx: Quit smoking. There are many programs available to help those who would like to quit, but you can get a head start with these do-it-yourself basics. To prepare yourself for quitting:

- Make a list of reasons to quit (kids, health, budget).
- List the immediate benefits (more stamina, less coughing, a sweeter-smelling house) and post it where you can see it many times a day.
- Make it public. Announce your intentions to those close to you. This signals commitment.
- Turn your goal into numbers, so it can be measured or charted—like the number of hours without a cigarette, the number of cigarettes smoked, or the number of dollars saved.
- Create a plan. Expect to feel nervous, anxious, and hungry—so . . .
- Choose the starting week carefully!
- Think of ways to keep your hands busy (yoga, sculpture, worry beads).
- Think of ways to keep your mouth busy (singing, carrot sticks, chewing gum).
- Think of ways to keep your brain busy (brisk walks, a new health-club membership, books on tape).

- Go to places where smoking is not allowed (libraries, movies, restaurants).
- Reward yourself for very small successes—it's difficult to wait until the first big one (points, stars, a CD, a new shower gel).

Rx for drinking: The biggest obstacle to kicking an alcohol habit is denial: denying the problem and denying the need for outside help. To assess the problem, ask yourself if drinking has interfered with your job, friendships, or family life for at least a month. If the answer is "yes," the diagnosis is alcohol abuse. If you have also built up a tolerance, need a drink to function adequately, or suffer from withdrawal when you try to stop, the diagnosis is alcohol dependence. Whether you drink every night, drink heavily only on weekends, or go on "benders" from time to time, the problem is still alcoholism, and you're not running your life—alcohol is! Though some people can get control of their drinking on their own, outside help may make it much easier to stick with sobriety when stress or disaster hits again.

Rx for drugs: If you feel insecure without a supply of your drug of choice or if you lie or feel guilty about your drug use, miss social occasions because of it, are spending too much time and money on it, have developed a tolerance to it, or sneak away from work or family to use it, you need help. As with alcohol, kicking a drug habit may go more smoothly with outside help. But you can try these suggestions first:

- Identify the emotions from which you're trying to escape—often loneliness, boredom, anger, or stress—and address them directly and constructively.
- Try going drug-free one day a week, then two, then more—until you're drug-free every day.
- Reward yourself with gifts or trips. (Using drugs less often means having more money!)

Rx for overeating: According to research done about ninety days after September 11, people eat more after a disaster. There are many reasons besides hunger: as a distraction from annoyance, worry, or loneliness; to delay doing something unpleasant; to fill up when empty of love, affection, or warmth; to find comfort with favorite foods; or to return to the good old days with old-fashioned or home-cooked food. If overeating is a personal problem, take a moment to look inside and see if you might be eating for emotional reasons. Once feelings are acknowledged and greeted, the desire to eat too much may fade; the following tricks can take you the rest of the way:

- Schedule snacks and meals.
- Eat snacks and meals at the table only.
- Make snacks and meals a feast for the eyes with pretty place mats, napkins, and glassware.
- Go low-fat and low-calorie.
- Drink lots of water.
- Exercise to control hunger.

Rx: Seek out the real fixes. If unhealthy quick fixes such as smoking, alcohol, drugs, and food have taken center stage in your life, it's time to put something else in the spotlight! After confronting the emotions, which are usually the main reason quick fixes tempt us, fill your life with *real* fixes that work, don't do damage, and support forward motion:

- Exercise.
- Do manual labor—gardening, carpentry, repairs.
- Take a walk with a child or dog and remind yourself what it's like to feel enthusiastic.
- Try a new skill.
- Share a project with a friend, such as making a quilt.
- Read.
- Pamper yourself.
- Clean out your wallet, drawer, or closet.
- Make a list.
- Watch cartoons.
- Do volunteer work.
- Write in your journal.
- Add some music to your life: listen, play, or sing.
- Get outside. Rake leaves or pot plants.
- Pray or meditate.

Rx: Get physical exercise. If you feel tired, lethargic, isolated, withdrawn, sleepless, or sexless, physical exercise can help get the body back on track. Exercise pumps up circulation, releases endorphins (the body's natural painkillers), and is an opportunity to get out and be with other people, even if it's just to run side by side on a treadmill. Morning exercise and grabbing daylight on cloudy and snowy days—even if it's just during lunch—will help reset your body's daily clock.

Rx: Head off PMS. Now that premenstrual syndrome is no longer considered a mental health issue, physicians and health-care professionals have become open to the idea that it may be correctable or at least modifiable and doing so is wise when disaster stress is threatening to drag you down. Among the prescriptions that physicians may recommend for some women are antiprostaglandins, tranquilizers, selective serotonin-reuptake inhibitors, calcium, progesterone, vitamin B6, diuretics, and bromocriptine (for breast tenderness). Home remedies include cutting back on salt intake to reduce water retention (don't overdo this in the summer) and aerobic exercise for thirty minutes a day, which fights depression and flushes extra fluid out of the body. Many women find that minor changes in diet make a big difference; eliminating alcohol and caffeine, for example, can reduce outbursts and irritability. An increase in carbohydrates may help to increase brain serotonin, which in turn may reduce depression, tension, anger, confusion, sadness, and fatigue, and increase alertness and calmness. Maybe this is why some of us crave carbohydrates premenstrually; we may be trying to self-medicate with potatoes, bread, pasta, cake, and candy! (Not the best way to go.) Six small meals rather than three big ones reduces hunger and prevents bingeing on sweets.

Rx: Head off menopause symptoms. If a disaster makes menopause symptoms more unbearable than they would ordinarily be, estrogen/progesterone replacement therapy may relieve the discomfort and may also slow osteoporosis. For women who are not candidates for hormone replacement therapy because of a history of breast cancer, blood clots, or other disorders, try topical solutions such as water-soluble jellies that relieve vaginal dryness. Consult your physician for more information.

Rx: Head off heart disease. If your cholesterol count climb, and blood flow dwindles, worrying about future heart attacks can add stress to stress and maybe even increase heart disease risk. Fortunately, there are a number of things people can do improve their risk profile. Among them:

- Change eating habits to reduce the intake of cholesterol and animal (saturated) fats, which seem to encourage the liver to produce cholesterol precursors. Cutting fat also cuts calories and leads to weight loss.
- Increase exercise to "use up" the noradrenaline, epinephrine, and fatty acids that pour into the bloodstream during stress. Exercise also cuts calories and leads to weight loss.
- Take medication to lower blood pressure or increase tranquility.
- Get diabetes under control.

PLAN AHEAD

Rx: Plan the anniversary. Although it's natural to dread any anniversary of a disaster great or small, to want to ignore it, planning for it allows you to take control and guide your emotions. Without a commemorative service or ritual as a focus, calls and words of sympathy may spread over weeks. If the tragedy was shared by a community or a nation, the memorials may stretch through too many excruciating days and nights. Paying your respects is healthy. Make sure to schedule some very private time to grieve. Anniversaries can be too big to bear unless there is planning.

Rx: Plan to accept anniversary emotions. When a disaster was a national experience, media rebroadcasts may stir up old hurts we thought were gone. Comments from well-meaning friends will bring back that out-of-control feeling . . . and our pain. Expect it all—let the feelings flow, and the tears, too, if they come. Expressing emotions is always the quickest way to move past them.

Rx: Watch for PTSD. Disaster pain normally recedes slowly as the years intercede. Thinking about the disaster, talking about it, and revisiting it help with the process of desensitization and integration. However, in a handful of cases—about one in twenty-five Americans—the pain evolves into Post-Traumatic Stress

Disorder. Symptoms of PTSD usually begin within three months of the traumatic event, but sometimes they don't show up for years. Symptoms include re-experiencing, avoidance, and heightened arousal (overreaction). If the trauma was sexual assault or childhood abuse, it's possible that major depression, social phobia, generalized anxiety, or panic attack will also appear. PTSD symptoms are particularly likely to appear during anniversaries of the disaster—or when the right cues are in place.

PTSD symptoms can persist for years if they go untreated and can place the sufferer in a worsening spiral of negative emotions and consequences, such as depression, drug abuse, alcohol abuse, eating disorders, and divorce. It's important to see a physician, psychologist, or psychiatrist if you suspect you have PTSD. Antidepressants, tranquilizers, desensitization therapy, cognitive behavior therapy, and stress management training can all help to turn PTSD symptoms around.

Rx: Inform your family and friends about the way you react. If you were blindsided by crying, hostility, depression, flashbacks, or similar phenomena on holidays or the last time an anniversary rolled around, it will help to be prepared next time. That includes telling loved ones what might be going on in your mind, so they'll understand—and treat you with compassion.

Where to Get Help for Post-Traumatic Stress Disorder

Information provided by the National Institute of Mental Health (NIMH)

To get a referral to a mental health professional in your local area or to obtain information on self-help groups and other resources located near you, contact the national mental health organizations listed below. Each group has developed its own procedures for referrals and has information on cities throughout the United States.

Following is a list of mental health organizations to help you find more information about anxiety disorders and related issues. NIMH is not responsible for the contents of any website listed.

American Academy of Child and Adolescent Psychiatry
3615 Wisconsin Ave., N.W.
Washington, D.C. 20016
(202) 966-7300
Internet: http://www.aacap.org
Call or write for referral information about child and adolescent psychiatrists in your area. (A child psychiatrist is a physician with five additional years of training beyond medical school in child, adolescent, and general psychiatry.)

American Counseling Association
801 N. Fairfax St., Suite 304
Alexandria, VA 22314
(800) 326-2642

Internet:
http://www.counseling.org
Call or write for referral information about counselors in your area.

American Psychiatric Association
Public Affairs Office, Suite 501
1400 K St., N.W.
Washington, D.C. 20005
(202) 682-6220
Internet: http://www.psych.org
For referral information about psychiatrists in your area, call or write the APA Public Affairs office.

American Psychological Association
750 First St., N.E.
Washington, D.C. 20002
(202) 336-5800
Internet: http://www.apa.org
Call or write for referral information about psychologists in your area.

Anxiety Disorders Association of America
11900 Parklawn Dr., Suite 100
Rockville, MD 20852-2624
(301) 231-9350
Internet: http://www.adaa.org/
Call or write to receive a list of mental health professionals who treat anxiety disorders and a list of self-help groups in your area. (Include $3.00 for postage and handling.)

Association for Advancement of Behavior Therapy
305 Seventh Ave., 16th Floor
New York, NY 10001
(212) 647-1890
Call or write AABT to request a list of mental health professionals in your state who use behavior therapy and/or cognitive behavior therapy—forms of treatment that are usually goal-oriented, short-term, and drug free. Sent with it is the brochure "Guidelines for Choosing a Behavior Therapist." AABT requests $5.00 to cover its postage and handling costs.

Freedom From Fear
308 Seaview Ave.
Staten Island, NY 10305
(718) 351-1717
Call or write for a free newsletter
on anxiety disorders and a referral list of treatment specialists.

**National Alliance for the
Mentally Ill**
200 N. Glebe Rd., Suite 1015
Arlington, VA 22201
(800) 950-NAMI
Internet: http://www.nami.org
For help in finding self-help
groups, NAMI can provide phone
numbers of state and regional
chapters and affiliates in your
area.

National Anxiety Foundation
3135 Custer Dr.
Lexington, KY 40517-4001
(606) 272-7166
NAF provides referrals to their
members and other mental health
professionals around the country.
(Include $10.00 for postage and
handling.)

**National Association of Social
Workers**
Clinical Registrar Office
750 First St., N.E., Suite 700
Washington, D.C. 20002-4241
(800) 638-8799
Internet: http://www.naswdc.org
Call or write for referrals to qual-
ified clinical social workers in
your area.

**National Depressive and
Manic-Depressive Association**
730 N. Franklin, Suite 501
Chicago, IL 60610
(800) 826-3632
Call or write for a list of support
groups in your area.

**National Mental Health
Association**
1021 Prince St.
Alexandria, VA 22314-2971
(703) 684-7722 or
(800) 969-NMHA
Internet: http://www.nmha.org
Call or write for a list of affiliate
mental health organizations in
your area who can provide

resources and information about self-help groups, treatment professionals, and community clinics. (Include $1.00 for postage and handling.)

National Panic/Anxiety Disorder News, Inc.

1718 Burgandy Pl.
Santa Rosa, CA 95403
(707) 527-5738
Internet:
http://www.npadnews.com
Call or write for referral sources and contacts for support groups for many parts of the country.

Obsessive Compulsive Foundation

9 Depot St.
Milford, CT 06460
(203) 878-5669
Internet: http://pages.prodigy.com/
alwillen/ocf.html
Call or write for a list of mental health practitioners in your area who specialize in treating OCD.

Additional Self-Help Groups

The following lay organizations can provide additional referral information on national and local self-help groups. Several also provide monthly publications as well as guidelines and materials for starting a self-help group.

ABIL, Inc.

(Agoraphobics Building Independent Lives)
3805 Cutshaw Ave., Suite 415
Richmond, VA 23230
(804) 353-3964
E-mail: ABIL1996@aol.com
Founded in 1986. National network of support groups.

A.I.M.

(Agoraphobics in Motion)
1719 Crooks St.
Royal Oak, MI 48067-1306
(248) 547-0400
E-mail: anny@ameritech.net
Founded in 1983
20 groups nationally

American Self-Help Clearinghouse
Northwest Covenant Medical Center
25 Pocono Rd.
Denville, NJ 07834
(800) 367-6724 (in NJ)
(201) 625-9565 (outside NJ)
Internet:
http://www.cmhc.com/selfhelp/
Founded in 1990
National network

National Mental Health Consumers' Self-Help Clearinghouse
1211 Chesnut St. Suite 1000
Philadelphia, PA 1910
(800) 553-4539 or
(215) 735-6082
Internet: http://www.libertynet.org/
~mha/cl_house.html
Founded in 1985
National network

Phobics Anonymous
P.O. Box 1180
Palm Springs, CA 92263

(619) 322-COPE
Founded in 1985
142 groups nationally

Recovery, Inc.
802 N. Dearborn St.
Chicago, IL 60610
(312) 337-5661
Founded in 1987
850 chapters nationally

Research Programs
The following institutions have treatment research programs and ongoing studies that are conducted with support from NIMH. Individuals with anxiety disorders, and their family members, may be eligible to participate in these studies.

University of California, Los Angeles
Anxiety Disorders Behavioral Program, Department of Psychology, Franz Hall
Room A225, 405 Hilgard Ave.
Los Angeles, CA 90095-1563
(310) 206-9191

NIMH Anxiety Disorders Clinic
National Institutes of Health
Clinical Center Building 10
4th Floor Outpatient Clinic
Bethesda, MD 20892-1368
(301) 496-4874

San Diego State University
Psychology Clinic
6363 Alvarado Ct. #103
San Diego, CA 92120
(619) 594-5134

The Johns Hopkins University
The Johns Hopkins Medical
Institutions Anxiety Disorders
Clinic
600 N. Wolfe St.
Meyer Room 115
Baltimore, MD 21287
(410) 955-5653

**Yale Anxiety Disorder
Research Center**
Connecticut Mental Health Center
34 Park St., Room 269
New Haven, CT 06519
(800) 538-0284 (in CT)
(203) 789-6985

Boston University
Center for Anxiety and Related
Disorders
648 Beacon St.,
6th Floor
Boston, MA 02215-2015
(617) 353-9610

**Yale University School of
Medicine**
West Haven VA Medical Center
Psychiatry
116A2 950 Campbell Ave.
West Haven, CT 06516
(203) 932-5711

Harvard University
Department of Psychology
33 Kirkland St.
Cambridge, MA 02138
(617) 495-3853

University of Florida
Center for the Study of Emotion
and Attention
P.O. Box 100165HSC
Gainesville, FL 32610
(352) 392-2439

University of Michigan
Anxiety Disorders Clinic Med.
Inn C435
1500 E. Medical Center Dr.
Ann Arbor, MI 48109-0840
(313) 764-5348

University of Iowa
Psychiatry Outpatient
University of Iowa Hospitals
and Clinics
200 Hawkins Dr.
Iowa City, IA 52242-1000
(319) 353-6314

Wayne State University
Depression/Schizophrenia/
Anxiety Studies
2751 E. Jefferson, Suite 200
Detroit, MI 48207
(313) 993-3426

University of Pittsburgh
Western Psychiatric Institute
and Clinic
Anxiety Disorders Clinic
3811 O'Hara St.
Pittsburgh, PA 15213-2593
(412) 624-1000

University of Nebraska, Lincoln
Psychological Consultation
Center
Department of Psychology
116 Lyman
Lincoln, NE 68588-0308
(402) 472-2351

Pennsylvania State University
Department of Psychology
The Stress and Anxiety Disorders
Institute
541 Moore Building
University Park, PA 16802
(814) 863-6019

Albert Einstein College of Medicine
Phobia, Stress, and Anxiety
Clinic
Long Island Jewish Medical
Center Hillside Hospital
75-59 263rd St.
Glen Oaks, NY 11004
(718) 470-8442

Brown University/Butler Hospital
700 Butler Dr., Duncan Building
Box G-BH
Providence, RI 02906
(401) 444-1900

Columbia University
New York State Psychiatric
Institute
722 W. 168th St.
New York, NY 1003

(212) 960-2442
(212) 960-2438
(212) 960-2367

Medical University of South Carolina
Department of Psychiatry and
Behavioral Sciences
Clinical Research Division
171 Ashley Ave.
Charleston, SC 29425
(800) 369-5472

Acknowledgments

This book is dedicated to all those who help me through disasters—great and small—from Day One to The One-Year Anniversary and beyond!

To everyone at Newmarket Press, especially my literary mentor Esther Margolis, Harry Burton, Keith Hollaman, Julia Moberg, Shannon Berning, Kathryn McHugh, Frank DeMaio, MaryJane DiMassi, Timothy Shaner, and Paul Sugarman.

To my colleagues at the Stress Program at Mount Sinai Medical Center in New York City, to Senior Vice President Dr. Gary Rosenberg for his common sense and uncommon wisdom, Dr. Ken Davis and Dr. Richard Berkowitz for their encouragement, and Dr. Sheldon Glabman for his constant friendship and constant support.

To my editor, researcher, and cheerleader Joan Lippert.

To my friends Dr. Gordon Ball, Dr. Natan Bar-Charma, Joan and Roy Benjamin, Mel Berger, Michael Braverman, Dr. Alan and Kira Copperman, Trey Farmer, George and Belinda Folsey, Dr. Constance Freeman, Roberta Gallagher, Dr. Alisan Goldfarb, Dr. Larry Grunfeld, Drs. Carroll and Joseph Hankin, Kate

Harrington, Dr. Jack and Stacy Hirshawitz, Ellen and Herb Klapper, Larry Kramer, Arlene and Allan Lazar, Donna Markowitz, John McTiernan, Judge Milton Mollen, Justin Moritt, Dr. Tanmoy Mukherjee, Edith O'Donnell, Meredith and Kory O'Donnell, Dr. Stephen Oswald, Gail Phillips, Raimonda Porter, Dr. Ben and Doris Sandler, Dr. Richard and Judy Saphir, George Simonton, Michael S.M. Tadross, Mikey T., Jr., Mary Turko, Sheri Weschler, and Dr. Ruth Westheimer, for their emotional backing.

To everyone at FoxNews Channel, especially Roger Ailes, Bill Shine, Kevin Magee, Matt Singerman, Ron Messer, Maria Donovan, Daniela Zivkovic, Amy Sohnen, Lauren Green, E.D. Donahey, Steve Doocey, Brian Kilmeade, Rachel McEntee, Erin Rider, Susan Wertheim, Noelle Inguagiato, and Gwen Marder.

To Dennis Bradford, for his artist's eye and generous heart.

And to my fabulous family, Dr. Roy Witkin, Laurie Witkin, Joshua and Nicole Restieri, Scott Witkin, Nikki Witkin and Brian Keldsen, Carol Fisher, Shelly, Jim, Bobby and Joey Fisher, Gretchen and Valerie Pauley, and Dr. George Coco Radovic.

And, as always, to my awesome daughter Kimberly, my brilliant son-in-law Travis Pauley, their spectacular son Jacob Glen Pauley, and my dear mother, Dr. Mildred Witkin—for always caring and always sharing...

About the Author

Georgia Witkin, Ph.D., one of the nation's foremost authorities on stress, is Director of The Stress Program at the Mount Sinai Medical Center in New York City, where she is an Assistant Clinical Professor of Psychiatry and Assistant Professor of Obstetrics, Gynecology, and Reproductive Sciences. She hosts *Beyond the News* on FoxNews Channel, and is the weekly lifestyle contributor to its *Fox and Friends* morning program. For many years, she was the health contributor to NBC NewsChannel 4. Dr. Witkin has also appeared as a guest expert on *Oprah, 20/20, CBS News, Imus in the Morning*, CNN, *The Today Show*, and more than 100 other programs. Her articles and quotes have appeared in *Readers Digest, Parade, Time, Family Circle, Newsweek, USA Today, Business Week*, and many others. She is the author of eight books about stress, including *The Male Stress Survival Guide* and *The Female Stress Survival Guide*. She lives in New York City.

Stress Management Books
Available from Newmarket Press

Ask for these titles at your local bookstore or use the coupon on the following page and enclose a check or money order payable to: Newmarket Press, 18 East 48th Street, New York, NY 10017.

StressRelief: Dealing with Disasters Great and Small—What to Expect and What to Do from Day One to Year One and Beyond
Georgia Witkin, Ph.D.

Organized by timeline, Dr. Witkin spells out the sequence of recovery after disaster—whether it is the events of September 11 or the loss of a loved one—and provides unique StressRelief Prescriptions for the emotional and physical fall-out of such a trauma. 240 pages.

The Female Stress Survival Guide:
Everything Women Need to Know, 3rd Edition
Georgia Witkin, Ph.D.

Updated to address 21st century concerns, Dr. Witkin reveals the secrets of successful stress management, and shows how to increase one's sense of control with proven physical and mental techniques and improved problem-solving skills. 336 pages.

(more titles on next page)

The Male Stress Survival Guide:
Everything Men Need to Know, 3rd Edition
Georgia Witkin, Ph.D.
Introduction by Jack Hirschowitz, M.D.

The director of the Stress Program at the Mount Sinai School of Medicine in New York helps men identify the areas where they are the most vulnerable to stress: body, career, and personal—includes practical strategies for reducing stress. 256 pages.

Discovering the Power of Self-Hypnosis—The Simple, Natural
Mind-Body Approach to Change and Healing, 2nd Edition
Stanley Fisher, Ph.D.
Foreword by Gail Sheehy

Featured in *Fast Company*, this expanded guide shows you how you can use this AMA-approved technique to alleviate such problems as insomnia, smoking, overeating, memory loss, pain, skin allergies, and fear of flying. 240 pages.

StressMap: Personal Diary Edition—The Ultimate Stress
Management, Self-Assessment, and Coping Guide,
Expanded Edition
Essi Systems
Foreword by Robert K. Cooper, Ph.D.

The only stress measurement tool that integrates all major stress research—medical, psychological, and interpersonal—into a revealing self-portrait of stress health. Includes a self-scoring questionnaire. 96 pages.

Please send me:

___ Copies of *StressRelief* @ $12.95 PB (ISBN 1-55704-529-1)
___ Copies of *The Female Stress Survival Guide* @ $14.95 PB
(1-55704-520-8)
___ Copies of *The Female Stress Survival Guide* @ $24.95 HC
(1-55704-415-5)
___ Copies of *The Male Stress Survival Guide* @ $14.95 PB
(1-55704-496-1)
___ Copies of *The Male Stress Survival Guide* @ $24.95 HC
(1-55704-519-4)
___ Copies of *Discovering the Power of Self-Hypnosis* $14.95 PB
(ISBN 1-55704-502-X)
___ Copies of *Discovering the Power of Self-Hypnosis* $24.95 HC
(1-55704-361-2)
___ Copies of *StressMap* $16.95 PB (1-55704-081-8)

For postage and handling, please add $3.50 for the first book and $1.00 for each additional book. Allow 4-6 weeks for delivery. Prices and availability subject to change.

I enclose check or money order payable to **Newmarket Press** in the amount of $_____.

Name: _____

Address: _____

City/State/Zip: _____

For discounts on orders of five or more copies or to get a catalog, contact Newmarket Press, Special Sales Department, 18 East 48th Street, New York, NY 10017; phone: (212) 832-3575 or 1-800-669-3903; fax: (212) 832-3629; or e-mail: sales@newmarketpress.com.